# Evaluating Theories of Language: Evidence from Disordered Communication

Edited by Barbara Dodd PhD, Ruth Campbell PhD
and Linda Worrall PhD

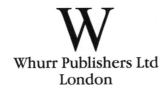

Whurr Publishers Ltd
London

**British Library Cataloguing in Publication Data**
A catalogue record for this book is available from the British Library.

ISBN 1-86156 000 1

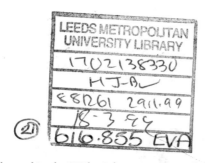
Printed and bound in the UK by Athenaeum Press Ltd, Gateshead, Tyne & Wear

# Contents

# Preface

Language is a specifically human accomplishment. As individuals, we are judged by how we communicate: what we say, how we say it and how we respond to what other people say. It is hardly surprising, then, that scholars have sought to understand how the human animal communicates. One approach to the study of language has been to investigate people whose ability to communicate is impaired. Researchers have argued that it is possible to identify the component mental processes that contribute to the ability to communicate by describing the ways in which language can break down in aphasia, or develop anomalously. Such impairments are not random and the constraints on the varieties of impairment might indicate the structural faultlines of language itself. Other researchers have expressed doubts about the extent to which data from impairment reflect normal language function. However, within each discipline studying language breakdown, there are specific questions to be addressed. As the number of disciplines and methodologies, and the sheer volume of data concerning language impairment multiply, we sometimes lose sight of important issues.

At most conferences there are groups of people muttering about the need to sit down for two days with a small number of people from a range of disciplines and discuss a single issue in depth. Our frustration with a standard conference led to a plan to hold a 'workshop' somewhere remote and beautiful. The theme was whether the study of individuals with impairment of communication clarified theory of normal function, and the extent to which theory of normal function had clinical application. This controversial issue had been addressed before, but seemed worthy of multidisciplinary re-examination. There were representatives from the disciplines of psycholinguistics, linguistics, neurophysiology and speech–language pathology from Australia, Britain, Hong Kong and the United States of America. Our aim was to take time to examine our basic assumptions about the relationship between data on communication disorder and theory of normal language function.

The World Health Organization (1980), in its *International Classification of Impairment, Disability and Handicap*, defines three aspects of communication disorder:

1.  *Impairment*, disturbance of structure or function, whether psychological, physiological or anatomical;
2.  *Disability*, the consequences of impairment for an individual in terms of functional or everyday performance or activity;
3.  *Handicap*, the disadvantage experienced by the individual due to impairment and disability, reflecting the value society attaches to disability.

The focus of the conference was at the level of impairment. Impairment includes the range of symptomatology that is associated with a disorder. As examples, people who have acquired brain injury may have deficits in language comprehension and production (aphasia); some children fail to acquire intelligible speech in the absence of any identified physical cause (developmental phonological disorder). While it is important to consider disability and handicap when planning intervention of a communication disorder, it is primarily data about impairment that is used to inform our understanding of normal communicative function.

This book presents a synthesis of a two day discussion where we explored the problems of constructing theory of how the normal brain deals with language using data from impaired individuals. The participants held different perspectives of impairment, influencing the questions they chose to address. Each of us presented a paper, which was discussed, rewritten, reviewed and modified. The end result appears here. The content includes theoretical reviews as well as new data. The foci of the participants' papers varied: critique of methodology; application of new technology; the study of bilingual people; and cross-linguistic studies. A range of language skills was discussed – phonology, prosody, syntax, semantics, reading and spelling. A range of developmental and acquired impairments was used as evidence – hearing impairment, cerebellar dysarthria, subcortical aphasia, cortical aphasia, phonological disorder, dyslexia. Initially some of us were a little bewildered by other participants' perspectives of areas we thought we understood clearly. Towards the end, what some had held as hard knowledge was transmuted to an assumption to be questioned.

# Acknowledgements

The editors wish to thank the contributors for their enthusiasm, willingness to engage in debate, and constructive review of their colleagues' chapters.

The contributors extend grateful thanks to Cathy Swart for compiling and formatting the book and keeping us to deadlines.

The publishers are grateful for permission to use the extracts printed on pages 37 and 51, from The Annotated Snark by Martin Gardner, which are reproduced with permission of Penguin Books Ltd and Simon Schuster, Inc.

Every effort has been made to obtain permission to reproduce copyright material throughout this book. If any proper acknowledgement has not yet been made, the copyright holder should contact the publisher.

# Contributors

**Andrew Butcher**
Flinders University, Adelaide, Australia
**Ruth Campbell**
Goldsmiths College, University of London, UK
**Max Coltheart**
Macquarie University, Sydney, Australia
**Barbara Dodd**
University of Newcastle, Newcastle-upon-Tyne, UK
**Michael Haller**
Macquarie University, Sydney, Australia
**Meredith Kennedy**
University of Newcastle, Newcastle-upon-Tyne, UK
**Leonard L. La Pointe**
Arizona State University, USA
**Robyn Langdon**
Macquarie University, Sydney, Australia
**Randi C. Martin**
Rice University, Texas, USA
**Paul F. McCormack**
Flinders University, Adelaide, Australia
**Bruce E. Murdoch**
University of Queensland, Brisbane, Australia
**Lydia So**
University of Hong Kong, Hong Kong
**Li Wei**
University of Newcastle, Newcastle-upon-Tyne, UK
**Linda Worrall**
University of Queensland, Brisbane, Australia
**Edwin M.-L. Yiu**
Curtin University, Perth, Australia

# Introduction
# Words and Nature

LEONARD L. LA POINTE

> In the world of words, the imagination is one of the forces of nature.
>
> Wallace Stevens

## Introduction

In July 1995 an international group of scholars on human communication and its disorders gathered for a workshop in a unique and magical setting to present papers, to react, to imagine, to engage in spirited discourse, to dissect complexities, and to attempt a strengthening of our grasp of a curious and paradoxical topic. The theme was the usefulness of analysis of the interactive nature of normal and impaired communication processes. Specifically, questions addressed the notions, can we use the data and tenets of what we know about normal processing to inform us about impaired processing. Conversely, and equally as intriguing to some, can we use the data and canons of impaired processing to nurture explanation of normal processes? This is a tantalising and confounding reversible issue that has not been unexplored in the past. Cognitive scientists, neuropsychologists, linguists, computational experts, behavioural neurologists, and speech–language pathologists have turned over these mossy rocks before, and the state of cognitive–linguistic science assures that we are a long way from heuristic satiation. Past investment of effort, however, does not dissuade us from further pursuit of explanation and understanding of matters that are substantial and befitting. So these topics were considered anew, with the insight and benefit of an accumulating archive of research on the theme. Nature facilitates creativity. Ample evidence abounds in the worlds of science, the humanities, and the arts that a strange amalgam of natural phenomena and human imagination can result in tangible harvest. So a setting was chosen to bring together words and nature. Experts who would study weighty issues on the relationship of impaired to normal communication processes juxtaposed against a natural backdrop of exquisite beauty. The

1

setting was O'Reilly's Rainforest Guesthouse in the Green Mountains, surrounded by the Lamington National Park up a scenic, serpentine road from Canungra, Queensland in Australia.

## Normal processes, impaired processes, models

As we shall see, and as others have indicated (Barsalou, 1992), the inter-play between data collection and theory development is often complex and multivariate. Cognitive psychologists and others interested in human communication and its disorders often disagree on the best ways for studying cognition and language. We should not be surprised by this disagreement, since the study of human cognitive–linguistic processes is such a diverse and enigmatic theme.

Additionally, cognitive and communicative science is still quite embryonic, or at best is in its infancy, relative to many other disciplines. We have not been around since the days of Hippocrates, Descartes, Flourens or Galen with subsequent centuries to bury our leeches and mistakes and cover our misdirection. Instead, our uncertainty and back-tracking, in the context of improved techno-availability of the archive of our art and science, is nearly immediately available for probing and dissection. Those who have studied the philosophy of science have commented regularly that revolution of scientific discovery appears to be much less common as an outcome than does cumulative evolution (Kuhn, 1970; McCauley, 1986; Bechtel, 1988; Barsalou, 1992). This flies in the face of popular wisdom and stereotype which appear to indicate that science develops in a logical, plodding, organised manner, and that each new discovery fits nicely into the puzzle of what has been previ-ously concluded. Common sense seems to indicate that scientists have a road map, and they know where they are going. Though Jay Rosenbek, (1995, personal communication) reminds us that 'common sense' is that sense that for centuries told us the world was flat.

Particularly in a new science, such as cognitive–communicative disor-ders, this view of the non-chaotic march of science is particularly fictional. Instead we pause, redo, reinvent, false start, explore redun-dantly, and occasionally break new ground. This is especially apparent in disciplines that do not have a clear general outline of a theory that will guide future research and that will persist for future theorists to articu-late in greater detail (Barsalou, 1992). So we struggle to see what we can learn. We grasp at insights. We view impairments to see if this suggests anything new about intact processes, and we wonder if a thorough explanation of normal processes will inform us about impairment or even better, guide us to a theory of therapy or intervention.

In aphasia, the aspect of cognitive and communicative impairment most familiar to me, the struggle over models, theory and treatment has intensified in recent years. Caramazza and his colleagues have written fairly extensively about what we can learn about normal cognitive structure from impaired performance as well as about theories of remediation of cognitive deficits (Rapp and Caramazza, 1991; Caramazza and Hillis, 1991). They remind us that inference about the structure of cognitive mechanisms from data derived from impaired subjects is problematic. One of the major problems centres on the complexity of inference in neuropsychology. As Rapp and Caramazza (1991) indicate, inferences about cognitive structure or psychological mechanisms is usually based upon sets of assumptions about the data that drive the inference.

It is very difficult to make one's assumptions explicit and even when the inter-nested assumptions are made explicit, researchers rarely seek independent confirmation of their validity. Conclusions, then, frequently are resting uncomfortably on a house of cards rather than a firm foundation. Rapp and Caramazza (1991) present several illustrative examples from the literature in neuropsychology that, in their opinion, rest on weak or unproven assumptions. If questions are raised about unreasonable conclusions from observed patterns of impairment, this clearly impacts on the interpretation of the relation of patterns of impaired or unimpaired performance.

Nevertheless, Caramazza and colleagues and others (Caramazza and Hillis, 1991; Gonzalez-Rothi and Moss, 1992; Byng, 1994; Hillis, 1993) have advocated or provided examples of model-based intervention strategies. Despite the problems involved in developing a science of model driven therapy, some writers appear optimistic that these obstacles can be worked through or around (Rapp and Caramazza, 1991). They point out that the considerable work in cognitive–communicative model building has had some concrete results. Firstly, and not unimportantly, especially in aphasia, models of processing in neuropsychology have increased our understanding of the disorders that occur as a result of brain damage. We are now able to specify more aptly and with greater confidence those mechanisms or processes that create the more global impairments. For example, instead of simply stating that an individual has impaired writing, Rapp and Caramazza (1991) indicate that now we may be able to explain further that the impaired writing is caused by inability to hold an orthographic representation in memory while motor commands for arm and hand movement are being assembled. These advances in understanding the nature of a deficit have also been apparent in the study of the reading process, with significant contributions by members of this conference. Testing empirically based architectural models of the normal language-processing system by careful exploration of whether or not damage to one of the components of these models could account for different disorders of language is the foundation of modern cognitive neuropsychology.

Byng (1994) reviews this approach and its influence or lack of influence in clinical aphasiology. These models offer a logical, sometimes even coherent, architectural framework for viewing language impairment, though the perils of oversimplified box-and-arrow diagrams are sometimes reminiscent of Radio Shack hard-wired diagrams of simple electronic devices rather than the multilevel, multiconnected, parallel-distributed reality of the complexity of the human nervous system.

Despite productivity in the arena of how cognitive neuropsychological models can advance our understanding of thinking about language as a number of processes and components, some of which can even be identified reliably across patients, some scholars in aphasia express reservations about the contributions of theory-driven therapy. Audrey Holland (1994), for example, states that the contributions that theory-driven therapy can make in the treatment of aphasia are limited in both number and scope. She suggests that most theories of cognitive processing are not theories about how to fix deficits; rather, they are theories about how and why the deficits occur.

Both Byng (1994) and Holland (1994) decry our lack of a coherent theory of therapy in aphasia (and this lament might well be raised in many other disorder areas of human cognitive–communicative dysfunction), and call for a focus of effort on the development of a such a theory of treatment. Byng (1994) gives several examples of how a theory of deficit is necessary for the development of a theory of therapy. She proposes that deficit analysis by itself is not enough to suggest formulation of specific therapeutic procedures. However, she advocates that analysis of the nature of the language impairment, rooted to a relationship of normal language processing, is a more informative way to construct therapeutic objectives and select remediation strategies.

Holland (1991), while being mindful of the limitations of cognitive neuropsychological theory to treatment in aphasia, is not unequivocal about the need to develop a richer conceptualisation of a theory of therapy. She states,

> If we are to serve aphasic patients better ... and turn clinical art into clinical science, then we must begin to develop explicit and falsifiable theories of treatment, to test their assumptions and contrast various theoretically-driven forms of treatment. (Holland, 1991)

Golper (1994), Byng (1994) and others echo these sentiments. Certainly we have not progressed to the point where a coherent theory of intervention or therapy can be assembled for all of the deficits seen in aphasia or in many of the other cognitive–communicative impairments, but it is clear that we can ill afford to be adrift on the clinical ocean without benefit of navigational guides. The navigational guides we possess at the moment might appear to be only stars and sextant, but nevertheless it would behove us to continue the voyage of trying to find out what we can learn from impairment about normal processing, as well as how normal processing can inform better understanding and management not only of impairment, but of the psychosocial aspects of disability and handicap created by cognitive–communicative disorders.

## Contributions at O'Reilly's

The impetus for this conference and subsequent book was generated in Brisbane at the University of Queensland, but subsequent contributions to the project were generated by scholars from London, Newcastle-upon-Tyne, Perth, Sydney, Adelaide, Brisbane, Hong Kong, Houston, and Tempe. As expected from consideration of a topic on which the universals have yet to be firmly entrenched, these contributions and the subsequent discussion generate a range of opinion. Strong support for the thesis that impairment can inform models of normal communication processes (and the converse) is apparent in some papers and healthy scepticism is conspicuous in others. Diversity in the pursuit of clarity is no vice.

Max Coltheart and his co-authors Robyn Langdon and Michael Haller advocate the contributions to models of language that are possible from the perspective of computational cognitive neuropsychology and acquired dyslexia. Coltheart and colleagues trace the rebirth some 40 years ago of flow-chart or box-and-arrow diagrams of cognitive psychology. While these authors give ample credit to other researchers for the 'rebirth' of cognitive psychology or the birth of cognitive neuropsychology, the contributions of Coltheart and a variety of colleagues certainly have had a presence in this birthing process as well. Coltheart's seminal contributions to the study of acquired dyslexia have a distinguished history in the development of how impaired language can inform aphasia theory and models of normal language. Now Coltheart and colleagues argue that it is time to evaluate critically the utility of computational cognitive neuropsychology in the development of models of language processing that can be artificially lesioned to test hypotheses about how people recognise printed words and read them aloud.

The wonderful or perhaps illusive world of prosody is visited by Paul McCormack, who queries 'Why are prosodic disorders so rare?' McCormack argues that the evidence is far from convincing that particular areas of the enchanted loom are responsible for specific aspects of prosodic functioning. The paper reviews data from studies of apraxia of speech, the dysarthrias, right hemisphere syndrome, and reports of 'foreign accent syndrome' and points out instances of obscured interpretation and conclusions regarding prosodic functioning and organisation.

Andrew Butcher takes a different tack in arguing against a model of gradual development and automatisation of motor programmes based on forms from the input lexicon. He asks 'how many lexicons?', and presents results from 'before and after' speech with postoperative cleft palate speakers and children with 'glue ear' after grommet insertion to show rapidity of acquisition of appropriate and consistent pronunciations. This, Butcher maintains, appears to be incompatible with the notion of gradual development of a separate output lexicon.

Ruth Campbell draws from another unique population to shed light on normal language and cognitive development. Campbell outlines some of the ways in which profound prelingual deafness impacts on language and cognition, particularly with the interactive variables of the role of Sign and lipreading. Campbell signifies the dynamic nature of deafness research, particularly regarding the influence of deaf culture on research agendas, and identifies several areas of study that may be fruitful in advancing our understanding of mechanisms and substrates of language. She indicates that careful exploration of the language and cognition of people who have been born deaf offers unrivalled opportunities for advancing theories of neural plasticity of cognitive–linguistic systems.

Professor Randi Martin discusses the issue of normal variation in cognitive architecture and the implications of these individual differences for neuropsychology. Martin argues that performance differences across normal subjects are entirely consistent with an analysis of a cognitive domain into components, and suggests that such differences make documentation of impairment more difficult though not impossible.

Barbara Dodd, Lydia H.K. So and Li Wei examine symptoms and signs of disorder in bilingual subjects who have atypical language learning experience but no specific type of impairment. From two experiments, one of phonological awareness in bilingual Chinese and English speaking university students and the second of phonological acquisitional errors in young bilingual speakers, Dodd, So and Wei argue that a particular language learning experience can lead to language behaviour in normal people that mimics impairment. Their findings support the view that differences in language behaviour may not necessarily reflect impairment of cognitive functions.

Bruce Murdoch traces the faint and hallowed steps of investigators and writers such as Luria as well as Penfield and Roberts when he visits the role of subcortical structures as a participant in language. Although the cerebral cortex has been regarded as the czar of language for generations, Murdoch points out that over the past two decades a proliferating number of clinico-neuroradiological studies have challenged the traditional view of the cerebral cortex as the sole neural province of language. Murdoch contends that advances in neuro-imaging and other windows to the brain, particularly the dynamic functional methods such as positron emission tomography (PET) and single photon emission computed tomography (SPECT), may be useful in drawing back the veil of uncertainty about the role of subcortical structures in language processing. Murdoch suggests that language compromise in subjects with lesions to the thalamus or striatum further lend evidence to models of subcortical participation in language.

Current research methodology in cognitive neuropsychology and aphasia is critically evaluated in the chapter by Meredith Kennedy. Kennedy holds that if the cognitive neuropsychological approach is to deal adequately with the intricacies of aphasia, replete with its complexity and variability, it may be appropriate to consider the extent to which other approaches to understanding aphasia either complement or supplant the cognitive neuropsychological approach. Kennedy raises questions about the sufficiency of double dissociations to contribute all we need to know about the nature of aphasic language impairment or models of single word processing in normal adults.

Edwin Yiu and Linda Worrall question the explanatory foundation of models of normal language processing and indicate that most studies of both normal and abnormal language processing are relatively Eurocentric. These authors point to cross-linguistic studies of sentence processing, particularly Cantonese, as instructive in testing the universality of language processing. Yiu and Worrall further highlight the existence of compensatory language functioning in aphasia as a complicating variable which must be considered in any model of impaired language processing that purports to inform normal language models.

## Dusk

Some issues and questions are arduous. Some phenomena blend and do not lend themselves to being dichotic or invariant. When, during twilight, does it become dark? Some propositions must be turned, considered and evaluated from varying perspectives and with accumulating evidence. Such may be the perplexity of the theme of this conference and book. These papers would suggest, however, that although the topic is fraught with complexity, we are developing paths of analysis that mark progress and occasional traces of consensus.

## References

Barsalou, L.W. (1992). *Cognitive Psychology: An Overview for Cognitive Scientists*. Hillsdale, NJ: Erlbaum Associates.

Bechtel, W. (1988). *Philosophy of Science: An Overview for Cognitive Science*. Hillsdale, NJ: Erlbaum Associates.

Byng, S. (1994). A theory of the deficit: A prerequisite for a theory of therapy? In M. Lemme (Ed.) *Clinical Aphasiology*, pp. 265–273. Austin, TX: Pro-Ed.

Caramazza, A. and Hillis, A. (1991). For a theory of remediation of cognitive deficits. *Reports of the Cognitive Neuropsychology Laboratory*. Baltimore: Johns Hopkins University.

Golper, L.C. (1994). Model-driven treatment: Promises and problems. In M. Lemme (Ed.) *Clinical Aphasiology*, pp. 283–289 Austin, TX: Pro-Ed.

Gonzalez-Rothi, L.J. and Moss, S. (1992). Alexia without agraphia: Potential for model assisted therapy. *Clinical Communication Disorders*, 2(1), 11–18.

Hillis, A.E. (1993). The role of models of language processing in rehabilitation of language impairments. *Aphasiology*, 7(1), 5–26.

Holland, A. (1991). *Some Thoughts on Future Needs and Directions for Research and Treatment of Aphasia*. National Institutes of Health.

Holland, A. (1994). Cognitive neuropsychological theory and treatment for aphasia: Exploring the strengths and limitations. In M. Lemme (Ed.) *Clinical Aphasiology*, pp. 275–282. Austin, TX: Pro-Ed.

Kuhn, T.S. (1970). *The Structure of Scientific Revolutions*, 2nd Edn. Chicago: University of Chicago Press.

McCauley, R.N. (1986). Intertheoretic relations and the future of psychology. *Philosophy of Science*, **53**, 177–199.

Rapp, B.C. and Caramazza, A. (1991). Cognitive neuropsychology: From impaired performance to normal cognitive structure. In R. Lister and H. Weingartner (Eds) *Perspectives on Cognitive Neuroscience*, pp. 384–403. Oxford: Oxford University Press.

# Chapter 1
# Computational Cognitive Neuropsychology and Acquired Dyslexia

MAX COLTHEART, ROBYN LANGDON AND MICHAEL HALLER

## Abstract

*Cognitive neuropsychology began with the study of reading, as a consequence of the seminal paper by Marshall and Newcombe in 1973 and subsequent work on acquired dyslexias over the next decade. In the 1980s the approach was extended to many other cognitive domains: spelling, the reception and production of spoken language, memory, visual agnosia and prosopagnosia, apraxia, and attentional disorders; and single case studies of treatment based on this approach began to appear.*

*An influential review of the field by Seidenberg (1988) complained that this work, while it had achieved much, had confined itself to considering the architecture of cognitive systems, and had said little or nothing about how the processing components of these systems actually worked. He argued that the time had come for cognitive modules to be computational – that is, to be expressed in the form of computer programs that actually performed the cognitive task in question. This endeavour forces modellers to be explicit about the way the processing components work. This is 'computational cognitive psychology'.*

*Such models can not only be used to explain facts about normal skilled reading; they can also be artificially lesioned in an attempt to simulate acquired disorders of cognition. This is 'computational cognitive neuropsychology'. Once again, it is reading that has been the initial domain of study. Two computational models of reading will be described, and attempts to explain detailed facts about surface and phonological dyslexia by appropriately lesioning these models will be presented and discussed.*

## Introduction

Cognitive psychology was reborn about forty years ago. Its reborn form had many new features, and one that was particularly distinctive was that theories about particular domains of cognitive processing were frequently expressed as flow-chart or box-and-arrow diagrams: Broadbent, Treisman, Neisser, Posner and Morton, and many others, chose this formalism to convey their theoretical ideas. There were several reasons for this, including a desire to be explicit (prose can hide things which flow-charts expose), the conception of cognition as information processing (so cognitive processing could be described as a sequence of operations by which representations were formed and transformed), and the computer model of mind (what a program does is describable in flow-chart terms, so what the mind does should also be so describable).

Nineteenth-century cognitive psychologists did not use diagrams like this; but nineteenth-century neurologists interested in the effects of brain damage upon cognition did. They were the so-called 'diagram-makers' such as Wernicke and Lichtheim. The boxes or 'centres' in these diagrams were meant to represent brain regions, and the arrows were meant to represent neural pathways, but since each centre had a particular cognitive function it was easy to read these diagrams as descriptive of the organisation of the mind rather than of the organisation of the brain.

The confluence of this nineteenth-century mode of neurology and the flow-chart formalism of modern cognitive psychology led to the development of cognitive neuropsychology. The first paper on the cognitive neuropsychology of reading (Marshall and Newcombe, 1973) not only described three different forms of acquired dyslexia, but also offered a model of reading expressed in flow-chart form, and an interpretation of each pattern of acquired dyslexia in terms of selective patterns of damage to specific components of the model. The cognitive neuropsychology of reading has adopted this approach ever since; and indeed it soon spread to the study of acquired dysgraphia, and then to work on many other forms of acquired impairment of cognition.

The achievements of cognitive neuropsychology, as surveyed in Ellis and Young (1988), Shallice (1988) and McCarthy and Warrington (1990), have been impressive and influential. Nevertheless, various authors have remarked upon certain limitations of the approach. Saffran (1982) for example argued that 'evidence from pathology may be more useful for the purpose (of) isolating cognitive subsystems and describing their general properties than in specifying how particular subsystems are utilised in the normal state'; and Shallice (1988) asserted that 'The most favourable level for effective mediations between neuropsychology and the theory of normal processing seems likely to be not that of the detailed operation of computational models, but that of the more global functional architecture'.

These issues were taken up in a particularly trenchant and thoughtful review of the state of cognitive neuropsychology by Seidenberg (1988). He reiterated the point that cognitive psychologists and cognitive neuropsychologists who were using modular models of cognition expressed in flow-chart form were only defining the architectures of these models; nothing was being said about how the processing components of the models actually worked, only about what these components were. To really understand cognition, Seidenberg argued, one needs to know how such components actually work. What Seidenberg was advocating was a move towards computational cognitive psychology. This way of doing cognitive psychology depends upon the flow-chart terminology for expressing theories about cognitive systems, but goes beyond it by requiring that these flow-charts be turned into actual working computer programs (such as the program he was currently working on, which became the computational model of reading described by Seidenberg and McClelland (1989)). The rise of connectionism in the 1980s gave great impetus to the view that cognitive psychology should become computational, and this view is now becoming widespread – for example, a number of computational models of reading have recently been developed (Reggia, Marsland and Berndt, 1988; Seidenberg and McClelland, 1989; Coltheart, Curtis, Atkins and Haller, 1993; Bullinaria, 1996; Zorzi, Houghton and Butterworth, 1995; Plaut, McClelland, Seidenberg and Patterson, 1995).

Why do this? The motivation has nothing to do with the computer model of mind. Any program which expresses a computational model is simply a tool, not a theory. It is a tool for detecting previously-unsuspected ambiguity, vagueness or inexplicitness in one's theories (it is not possible to express a modular model as a modular computer program that actually runs, without specifying exactly how each module does its particular information-processing job); and also a tool allowing far more rigorous theory testing. The flow-chart approach had both of these virtues; the computational approach just does both jobs better (Coltheart, 1994) – which is why a wholesale move by cognitive psychologists towards computational modelling of cognition would seem a good idea.

Computational cognitive psychology is thus an approach to studying cognition in which any theory about the nature of cognitive processing in some domain – face recognition, working memory, inference-making, for example – is expressed in the form of a computer program that actually carries out the cognitive activity in question - the program actually recognises faces, or stores and retrieves information from a working memory, or draws inferences. The theorist's claim is that the way the program does the job is also the way that people do it; and a rigorous test of this claim is to determine whether the variables that affect a human subject's speed or accuracy affect the program's speed or accuracy in the same way.

Just as there is a subfield of cognitive psychology known as cognitive neuropsychology, so a subfield of computational cognitive psychology is developing – computational cognitive neuropsychology. What this does is to take computational models of cognition and test them by investigating whether one can reproduce various forms of acquired disorders of cognition by 'lesioning' the model – deleting some of its processing units, cutting some of its connections, adding noise to some of its computations. Can one create a lesioned model whose behaviour matches in detail the behaviours of particular patients with acquired disorders of the relevant domain of cognition? The closer such matches are, the more confidence one will have in the theory of normal cognition embodied in the computational model.

In this chapter, we consider work on the computational cognitive neuropsychology of reading. Some domains of cognition have no computational models yet; however, the domain of reading, as mentioned above, has several. Two of these models of reading, the Dual-Route Cascaded (DRC) model (Coltheart et al., 1993; Coltheart and Rastle, 1994) and a parallel-distributed-processing model (Plaut et al., 1995) have been applied to the simulation of several forms of acquired dyslexia; so in this chapter we will focus on these two computational models. Evidence from acquired dyslexia is currently critical for adjudication between the competing theories of reading that generated these computational models.

## Computational modelling of reading

### The Seidenberg and McClelland (1989) model

In this model, which we will refer to as the SM model, there were two routes from print to speech, but only one was actually implemented in the computational form of the model. The unimplemented route was an indirect pathway which went from print to meaning and then from meaning to speech. Since it was not implemented, it played no role in the model's simulations of results from studies of normal reading and acquired dyslexia. What was important here was the implemented pathway, which was a pathway that went directly from print to speech without any intervening level of representation; and what was critical about this pathway was the claim that it was capable of correct reading aloud for both exception words and nonwords. Previously, it had been argued that no single procedure for reading aloud could correctly read these two types of letter string. Exception words, since they disobey grapheme–phoneme rules, must be read aloud by recourse to word-specific knowledge about print-to-speech relationships ('lexical reading'). Nonwords, since they by definition cannot have recourse to word-specific knowledge, must be read aloud by recourse to a system of general rules about the mappings of graphemes to phonemes ('non-lexical reading'). This claim was directly confronted by Seidenberg and McClelland (1989).

This theoretical claim about the impossibility of a single procedure that could correctly read aloud both exception words and nonwords had always been bolstered by two forms of empirical data: one concerning effects of exceptionality of grapheme–phoneme correspondences on normal subjects' naming latencies, and the other concerning the contrast between two forms of acquired dyslexia, surface dyslexia and phonological dyslexia.

Many studies of normal readers (e.g. Seidenberg, Waters, Barnes and Tanenhaus, 1984; Taraban and McClelland, 1987; Paap and Noel, 1991) have shown that naming latencies for exception words are longer than naming latencies for regular words, but only when the words are of low frequency. Traditionally, this had been interpreted as follows: the lexical and non-lexical ways of reading aloud will produce the same response to a regular word, but conflicting responses to an exception word, and this conflict will lengthen the naming latency. The conflict does not affect performance with high-frequency words because the lexical route is sensitive to word frequency to such a degree that non-lexical processing is too slow to influence performance with high frequency words. The results with low-frequency words were taken as strong evidence for the idea that there are distinct lexical and non-lexical reading-aloud mechanisms. However, reading by the implemented route of the SM model, a route which does not embody such a distinction, was also sensitive to the exception/regular distinction, and the size of the exception effect was greater for low-frequency words.

What of the second form of empirical data, the results from acquired dyslexia? Since Seidenberg and McClelland wished to show that the evidence previously taken as favouring the lexical route/non-lexical route distinction did not in fact require such a distinction, they also considered whether there were ways in which they might simulate forms of acquired dyslexia by artificially lesioning their model. Patterson, Seidenberg and McClelland (1989) and Patterson (1990) report results from studies in which the implemented route of the SM model was damaged in various ways (e.g. by adding noise to its computations, or by deleting processing units) to try to generate a damaged system in which nonwords and regular words were read better than exception words (this is surface dyslexia). As for phonological dyslexia, where words are read well and nonwords badly, Seidenberg and McClelland proposed (p. 558) that this would follow if the patient's capacity to compute pronunciations from print were impaired but the indirect route from orthography to meaning to phonology were not – that is, phonological dyslexia is reading via meaning.

## Criticisms of the Seidenberg and McClelland model

### (a) Nonword reading by the SM model

Although Seidenberg and McClelland suggested that the implemented route of their model could read exception words and nonwords as well as normal readers can, this turned out not to be the case. Exception word reading by the model was certainly very accurate, but nonword reading was not: analyses of the nonword reading performance of the SM model by Besner, Twilley, McCann and Seergobin (1990) showed that its percentage correct was far lower in this task than that shown by normal readers.

### (b) The SM model's account of acquired dyslexias

As far as surface dyslexia is concerned, Coltheart, Curtis, Atkins and Haller (1993) pointed out that the attempts to simulate this pattern of acquired dyslexia by lesioning the SM model in various ways had not been successful. These attempts had used data from two particularly pure surface dyslexic patients, MP (Bub, Cancelliere and Kertesz, 1985) and a more severe case KT (McCarthy and Warrington, 1986). Although it was possible to lesion the SM model so that its accuracy in reading regular and exception words was similar to the accuracy shown by MP, the lesioned model did not produce regularisation errors to a significant degree when it misread exception words, whereas MP almost always did; and no way could be found to lesion the model so that its accuracy with regular and exception words was similar to the accuracies shown by the patient KT.

As for phonological dyslexia, Coltheart et al. (1993) disputed the idea that the advantage of word reading over nonword reading in phonological dyslexia arose because these patients were reading words via meaning, on the ground that in some cases of patients with severe semantic impairments one saw very good word reading in the presence of abolished nonword reading (Funnell, 1983) and in others very good reading of exception words (Schwartz, Marin and Saffran, 1979). If the route that is used for nonword reading is abolished (as in the case reported by Funnell, 1983) then according to the SM model reading must be semantically mediated. Therefore, where there is severe semantic damage, word reading would have to be severely impaired too, and would have to show evidence of semantic effects (such as semantic errors, or a difference between performance with concrete words and performance with abstract words) – which was not so in the cases reported by Funnell (1983) and Schwartz et al. (1979).

In sum, then, the two traditional claims that no system lacking the distinction between a lexical and a non-lexical reading route could explain (a) how both exception words and nonwords are read aloud correctly, nor (b) how surface and phonological dyslexia arise, survived the challenge of the work by Seidenberg and McClelland (1989).

### The Plaut, McClelland, Seidenberg and Patterson (1995) model

Seidenberg, McClelland and colleagues responded to these criticisms of the SM model by developing a different though related model of reading aloud, which we will refer to as the PMSP model. It resembles the SM model in that it has an (unimplemented) route that goes from print via meaning to speech, and an implemented route that goes directly from print to speech. The implemented route has the same network architecture as the SM model had: an array of orthographic input units, fully connected to an array of hidden units, which in turn are fully connected to an array of phonological output units. Both models were trained to learn to read by some form of the back-propagation learning algorithm. Where the models differ is in the nature of the input units and the output units.

In the SM model, a letter in a visual stimulus had a distributed representation, in the sense that several different input units would respond to any one letter, and in the sense that any one input unit would respond to several different letters. Each input unit in the SM model was responsive to 100 different three-letter sequences, so a D in the input might excite one unit sensitive to the sequence ADG, another sensitive to the sequence BAD, and another sensitive to the sequence DGE, for example. Units at the phonological output level also generated distributed representations in a similar way: since each such unit stood for a particular ordered sequence of three phonetic features, any particular phoneme would excite a number of different output units, and any particular output unit would be responsive to a number of different phonemes.

In contrast, the PMSP model uses local representations at both the input and the output level. Importantly, the input units do not represent individual letters, but, in general, individual graphemes (where 'grapheme' means 'letter or letter group corresponding to a phoneme'). So, for example, there is an input unit for the grapheme FF and one for the grapheme TCH. Representations at the output level are also local: each unit at this level represents a particular phoneme, and any particular phoneme excites just one unit.

The tricky job of converting a string of letters to a string of graphemes is not performed by the model; the input submitted to the model is already coded as a set of graphemes. Thus what the model has to learn is not a conversion which is sometimes many-to-one (the translation of a letter string to a phoneme string, a conversion which is many-to-one for any letter string in which a phoneme is represented by more than one letter), but a conversion which is invariably one-to-one (the translation of a grapheme string to a phoneme string).

The PMSP model succeeds in reading nonwords at the level of accuracy shown by normal human readers. That is, after being trained on a corpus of about 3,000 words, roughly 22% of which are exception words, it correctly reads virtually all of a set of nonwords, none of which were in its training corpus, and most of which contain grapheme–phoneme correspondences which are contradicted by correspondences present in some of the exception words in the training corpus. Thus one of the two general criticisms of the SM model – its inadequacy in nonword reading - cannot be raised against the PMSP model. What of the other criticism, the inability to account for acquired dyslexias? We consider this question below. Before doing so, however, it is necessary to describe an alternative computational model of reading, the DRC ('Dual-Route Cascaded') model, which is also intended to be able to give an account of acquired dyslexias, since our aim is to compare the success with which each model can account for such dyslexias.

## The DRC model

At some points above we referred to traditional ideas about reading aloud involving the distinction between lexical (word-specific) and non-lexical (rule-based) procedures for reading aloud. The DRC model (Coltheart et al., 1993; Coltheart and Rastle, 1994) is a computational realisation of such ideas – in other words, it is a computer program that reads aloud using simultaneously a lexical lookup procedure and a GPC rule-application procedure.

The general architecture of the model is as shown in Figure 1.1. This architecture is essentially identical to the architecture of previous non-computational versions of the dual-route model of reading such as those in Coltheart (1985), Patterson and Shewell (1987) and Ellis and Young (1988). There is a rule-based GPC route for converting print to speech, which yields correct responses for all nonwords and regular words and regularisation errors for all exception words; and there is a lexical route, which yields correct responses for all words but cannot read any nonwords correctly.

This lexical route is divided into two subroutes. Once a word's representation in the orthographic input lexicon is accessed, there is a direct link to its pronunciation in the phonological output lexicon (the 'lexical/non-semantic route'), and also this output representation can be accessed indirectly, via the word's representation in the semantic system ('the lexical/semantic route').

The computational architecture of the model is shown in Figure 1.2. This is the architecture of the computer program derived from the general architecture of Figure 1.1.

The vocabulary of the model is all the monosyllabic words in the CELEX database (Baayen, Piepenbrock and van Rijn, 1993) – 7,991 words. The longest such word has eight letters. Hence the model has eight sets of letter detectors (one set for each possible position in the input string), and eight corresponding sets of feature detectors. When a letter string is presented to the model to be read aloud, it is initially represented at the feature level. All the features possessed by the first letter in the input string switch on their feature units in the first set of feature units; similarly for the second letter and the second set of feature units, and so on.

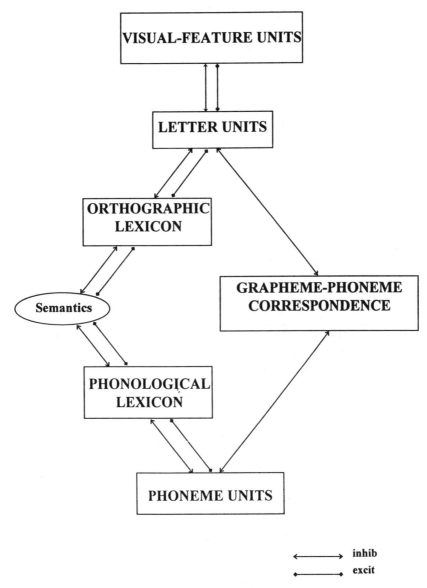

**Figure 1.1** General architecture of the DRC model.

All the feature units in the first set are connected to all the letter units in the first set. Feature units have excitatory connections to the units for letters that have those features, and inhibitory connections to letters that do not. So, for example, the feature 'Vertical on the left' excites such letter units as B D E and F and inhibits such letter units as A C and G.

Connections exist in both directions (the principle of 'interactive activation'), so that the letter unit for A excites such features as 'Horizontal in the middle' and inhibits such feature units as 'Vertical on the left' and 'Curve on the right'.

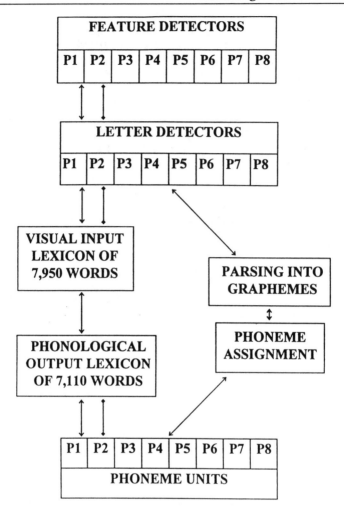

**Computational architecture of the DRC model**

```
•————————→• inhib
←————————→ excit
```

**Figure 1.2** Computational architecture of the DRC model.

The same kind of connectivity exists between the letter level and the orthographic input lexicon. Hence the unit for the letter C in the first set of letter units has an excitatory connection to every unit in the orthographic input lexicon representing a word beginning with C, and an inhibitory connection to every other unit, i.e. every unit representing a word that begins with any other letter. In the other direction, the unit for the word CAT in the orthographic input lexicon has an excitatory connection to the letter unit for C in the first set of letter units, and an inhibitory connection to all other units in that set.

A critical consequence of this connectivity scheme is that any letter string presented will excite a number of word units in the orthographic input lexicon to varying degrees. For example, the stimulus BAD could produce a small amount of activation in the word unit for PEN (the letter input B activates the feature 'Vertical on left' which produces some response in the letter unit P; the letter input A excites the feature 'Horizontal in the middle' which excites the letter unit E; and the letter input D excites 'Vertical on the left' which excites the letter unit for N). Of course, BAD will excite BAD much more than it will excite PEN, because there will be some inhibitory effects of the letter string BAD on the word unit for PEN but no such effects on the word unit for BAD. However, to sharpen the response of the orthographic input lexicon, every word unit in it has an inhibitory connection to every other word unit. So BAD and PEN will inhibit each other; and since BAD will be more strongly activated than PEN when the input is BAD, the BAD unit will reduce the activation of the PEN unit more than vice versa. Hence the difference in activation levels of the two units will widen as processing proceeds.

Each unit in the orthographic input lexicon has a direct excitatory connection to its representation in the phonological output lexicon. In turn there are connections from the phonological output lexicon to the phoneme level (and also inhibitory connections within the phonological output lexicon between every pair of units). Because no word in DRC's monosyllabic vocabulary has more than seven phonemes, there are seven sets of phonemes in the phoneme level. The unit for the word 'CAT' in the phonological output lexicon has an excitatory link to the phoneme unit /k/ in the first set of phoneme units, and inhibitory links to all other phoneme units in that set; similarly with the links to appropriate and inappropriate phonemes in the second and third phoneme sets. And there are analogous connections back from phoneme level to phonological output lexicon, so that the phoneme unit for /k/ in the first phoneme set has excitatory connections to all words in the phonological output lexicon that begin with that phoneme, and has inhibitory links to all words that begin with any other phoneme.

Some preliminary work (Patel and Coltheart, 1996) has begun on implementing a system of semantic representations with connections to and from the orthographic input lexicon and also to and from the phonological output lexicon; but this has not yet reached a stage where a semantic component can be added to the full DRC model.

That is how the lexical route of the DRC model works. There is also a non-lexical route which operates in parallel with the lexical route. The two routes share a common input system (the letter level) and a common output system (the phoneme level) but communicate between these levels separately. The non-lexical route has a graphemic parsing system which translates the letter string into a grapheme string, and a system of grapheme–phoneme correspondences which is applied to the grapheme string. This operates from left to right across the letter string. As each grapheme is converted to a phoneme, the representation of that phoneme in the appropriate set of phoneme units at the phoneme level begins to receive some activation.

Thus the phoneme units at the phoneme level receive activation from two sources. When the input is a regular word, these two sources contribute coherent information; when the input is an exception word, there will be some conflict between the information coming form the two sources.

This model succeeds in simulating a large range of results from experiments on lexical decision, reading aloud and priming in normal subjects (Coltheart et al., 1993; Coltheart and Rastle, 1994; Coltheart, 1995), but here we consider only attempts to use this model to simulate forms of acquired dyslexia, and comparison between these attempts and attempts to simulate acquired dyslexias using the competing computational model of reading, the PMSP model described above.

# Computational modelling of acquired dyslexias

In the past few years, there has been a considerable amount of work on computational modelling of a wide variety of acquired dyslexias, including deep dyslexia (Plaut and Shallice, 1993) and neglect dyslexia (Mozer and Behrmann, 1990). This work has not been in the context of models that have also been applied to the simulation of a variety of results from experiments with normal subjects, however, and so we will not consider it here, focusing instead upon three patterns of acquired dyslexia which have been considered in relation to both the PMSP model and the DRC model.

### Acquired dyslexias and the PMSP model

*(a) Surface dyslexia*

Attempts to simulate surface dyslexia have focused on two particularly pure cases, MP (Bub et al., 1985) and KT (McCarthy and Warrington, 1986). These cases are pure in the sense that nonword reading and regular word reading were essentially normal in both patients, whilst the ability to read exception words was markedly compromised, especially for low-frequency exception words. The cases are also pure in another sense – virtually every incorrect response to an exception word was a regularisation error (reading the word according to GPC rules). Data obtained from these two patients (as summarised in Plaut et al., 1995) are shown in Figures 1.3 and 1.4.

Both the intact PMSP model and the intact DRC model read aloud correctly all of these types of words and nonwords. The simulation task is

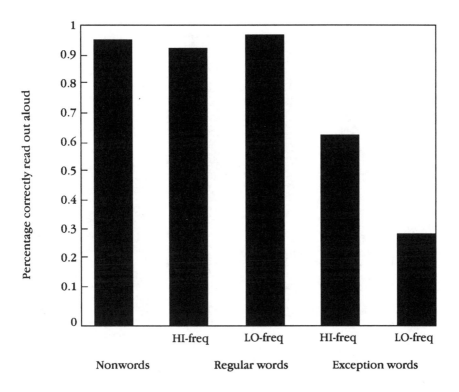

**Figure 1.3** Reading aloud in surface dyslexia: patient MP.

a daunting one: how to damage a model so as to leave intact its ability to read nonwords and regular words, whilst causing it to make errors in reading high-frequency exception words, and even more errors with low-frequency exception words. Indeed, the simulation task is even more daunting: because MP and KT almost always produced a regularisation error when they misread an exception word, almost all of the lesioned models' errors will have to be regularisation errors too. Finally, although both patients show exactly the same pattern of performance across the different stimulus types, KT shows a more extreme pattern than MP: can this severity effect be modelled by using different severities of lesion?

Patterson, Seidenberg and McClelland (1989) and Plaut et al. (1995) both found that lesioning the direct route of the SM or PSMP models could not yield a satisfactory simulation of surface dyslexia. So Plaut et al. adopted a different approach, following Shallice, Warrington and McCarthy(1983) in arguing that surface dyslexia arises when there is a disturbance of the semantic reading pathway (indeed, for a time Shallice and colleagues even called surface dyslexia 'reading without semantics'). Plaut et al. (1995) therefore wished to simulate surface dyslexia by lesioning the semantic route of their model, leaving the model to read as best it could by means of its direct route from orthography to phonology.

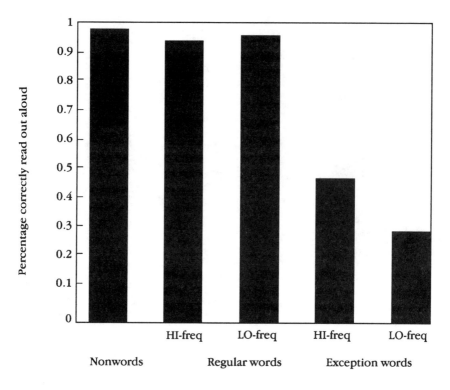

**Figure 1.4** Reading aloud in surface dyslexia: patient KT.

The first problem to deal with here is that there is no semantic route to lesion in the model, because the route from orthography to phonology via meaning is not implemented in the PMSP model, and implementation of it would be a massive endeavour: 'Including a full implementation of the semantic pathway is of course beyond the scope of the present work' (Plaut et al., 1995). Hence the semantic pathway was created artificially: the direct route of the model was trained to associate orthography with phonology in the usual way, but also, on each training trial, all output phonemes for that word were provided with external input (that is, input by the modellers, not by the model) that pushed these phoneme units towards their correct states (0 or 1). This phonemic input was meant to mimic input from a semantic system to the phonological output system

The second problem that had to be dealt with was as follows: one of the most important properties of the direct route from orthography to phonology in the PMSP model is that it is perfect at reading both exception words and nonwords. Indeed, Plaut et al. stress this at several points, emphasising its importance as a refutation of previous claims that no single procedure could read both types of stimuli, and also its importance as an advance beyond the SM model, whose direct route was meant to but could not read nonwords at a normal level.

But if this direct route reads all exception words correctly, then even if the semantic route were first implemented and then completely removed, the model would not be surface dyslexic. On the contrary, it would read all exception words flawlessly. What could be done about this? Plaut and colleagues approached this issue by developing a type of training regime which had the effect of preventing the direct route from learning all exception words, particularly low-frequency exception words.

This was done by making the amount of phoneme activation provided 'externally' on each training trial proportional to the frequency of the word presented on that trial and to the training epoch number. The effect of this procedure was that, after extended training, 'as the semantic pathway gains in competence, the phonological pathway increasingly specialises for consistent spelling-sound correspondences at the expense of exception words' (Plaut et al., 1995), particularly at the expense of low-frequency exception words. After this training regime, the 'semantic' route was deleted (that is, the phonological output system was deprived of the external input to correct phonemes that mimicked input from a semantic system) so that this 'semantically-lesioned' model was now reading only by its intact direct orthography-phonology route. This lesioned model did read regular words and nonwords correctly, and did misread some exception words, especially low-frequency ones. Thus the surface-dyslexic pattern seen in Figures 1.3 and 1.4 was successfully reproduced.

The severity issue remained a problem. Plaut et al. (1995) argue that the semantic route was damaged so much in both patients that all their reading aloud was accomplished by the direct route. Why, then, was MP more successful than KT at reading exception words, if both had the same lesion (complete removal of semantic contribution to reading aloud), and how could this difference between patients be simulated?

This was done by varying the number of epochs for which the network was trained before it was lesioned. With 400 training epochs, the reliance on the 'semantic' pathway is not yet very great, so the direct pathway is still fairly competent at reading low-frequency exception words. With 2,000 training epochs, the system has come to rely much more on the 'semantic' pathway, so the direct pathway now is much less competent at reading these low-frequency exception words. So stopping training after 400 epochs and lesioning the model by deleting the semantic contribution will produce less disastrous effects upon exception word reading - that is, a milder form of surface dyslexia – than will allowing training to proceed for 2,000 epochs before lesioning the model. A model trained for 400 epochs and then lesioned produced per cent correct reading rates with high and with low-frequency exception words that were very close to the values for MP's reading of such items. A model trained for 2,000 epochs and then lesioned produced per cent correct reading rates with high and with low frequency exception words that were very close to the values for KT's reading of such items.

The claim here is that MP's premorbid reading system must have been like one trained for only 400 epochs, whereas KT's must have been like one trained for 2,000 epochs. Unless this is to be a purely arbitrary claim, it needs some justification, and this was provided by the suggestion (Plaut et al., 1995) that 'differences amongst patients may not reflect differences in the severities of their brain damage. Rather, they may reflect differences in their premorbid reading experience, with the patients exhibiting the more severe impairment having the greatest premorbid reading competence . . . Note that we are assuming that KT had greater reading experience than MP; while there is no direct evidence on this issue, it is broadly consistent with the observation that KT was a college-educated banker (Shallice et al., 1983) while MP was educated only through high school)'. The idea here is that the more literate a normal reader is, the more reading aloud will use contributions from the semantic route. This will mean that the frequency cutoff below which the direct route cannot read exception words will be higher the more literate the reader. KT was more educated than MP, so, when both have to read via the direct route, KT will begin to fail with exception words at a higher frequency level than MP - which is what can be seen in Figures 1.3 and 1.4.

Thus the model which Plaut et al. (1995) obtained on the basis of these simulations of acquired dyslexia, a model partly computational and partly not, has two reading routes which have the following features: there is an indirect (semantic) route which can read all words but no nonwords, and there is a direct reading route which correctly reads all regular words and all nonwords, but which only reads exception words correctly when these are high in frequency. Level of literacy determines the competence of this route with exception words: the more reading experience a person (or the network) has, the poorer the direct route is at reading exception words.

It remains to be seen, as Plaut et al. (1995) acknowledge, whether after a genuine implementation of the semantic route, i.e. the construction of a fully computational model, the model would behave in this way after a semantic lesion. It is also worth noting that two of the important departures from the SM model introduced by Plaut et al. – the introduction of the grapheme as a unit, and the introduction of a pathway that reads regular words and nonwords well but regularises some, perhaps many, exception words – represent a substantial shift towards the traditional form of dual-route model (Coltheart, 1978).

More important, however, is the question of whether the model developed so as to simulate surface dyslexia is capable of simulating the other two forms of acquired dyslexia considered by Plaut et al. (1995) – namely, phonological dyslexia and lexical non-semantic reading.

## (b) Phonological dyslexia

In this form of acquired dyslexia, words are read relatively well (regardless of whether they are regular words or exceptions) and nonwords are read poorly. In the most extreme case (Funnell, 1983), nonword reading was completely abolished (0% correct), with word reading close to being intact (about 90% correct even for long abstract low-frequency words). Other cases are less extreme – for example, LB (Derouesne and Beauvois, 1985) could read about 50% of nonwords correctly (this varied with type of nonword – see below for further discussion).

According to both Seidenberg and McClelland (1989) and Plaut et al. (1995), phonological dyslexia in one of its forms involves reliance to a greater or lesser extent upon reading via meaning – that is, one way in which phonological dyslexia will occur is when a lesion of the direct route of their models forces the system to rely more than usual, or even entirely, upon the semantic reading route, which of course cannot read nonwords. They suggest this analysis for WB, the case of phonological dyslexia reported by Funnell (1983).

However, WB was not only phonological-dyslexic but also had a clear semantic impairment. When his ability to understand spoken words, pictures, or printed words was tested, a very marked impairment of the semantic system was evident, with confusions between semantically related items such as spoon/fork, orange/lemon, and bus/bicycle. Semantic errors also occurred frequently in picture naming. If he were relying to a substantial extent upon reading via semantics, semantic effects (such as semantic errors) should have been evident in his word reading, and such effects were minimal – his word reading was very good, with very few unambiguous semantic errors. Coltheart et al. (1993) and others regard this as one of the lines of evidence for the existence of a third reading route which is lexical (it can only read words) but not semantic (it does not involve semantic access, but instead uses a direct pathway from the orthographic input lexicon to the phonological output lexicon). Such a pathway is, of course, not present in the SM and PMSP models.

Plaut et al. (1995) have responded to such arguments by proposing that WB achieved word reading via the joint use of two partially impaired pathways, the semantic and direct pathways of their model. Neither pathway alone would do a good job of reading, but the two sources of partial information about words, one semantic and the other phonological, combine to support word reading (but not nonword reading, since semantic support is not available there).

The idea is that WB avoided making frequent semantic errors in reading aloud despite his semantic impairment, not by using a third reading route, but by blocking these errors using some phonological information derived from the direct phonological reading route. For example, WB when attempting to read the word orange might, because of his semantic impairment, be unsure whether it is that word or the word lemon – but just a single phoneme delivered from the direct route would allow him to make the correct choice between these two alternatives, and so avoid the potential semantic error.

But this argument requires that WB did have some partial ability to use this direct route, rather than complete abolition of it - and there was absolutely no evidence for such partial ability in WB. He not only scored 0% on nonword reading,[1] he scored 0% on sounding out single printed letters (even though he could repeat letter-sounds, and name single printed letters). If this is not accepted as evidence for complete abolition of this route, it is hard to see what would be.

We claim therefore that WB could not have been reading in the way proposed by Plaut et al., and hence that the data obtained with this particular case of phonological dyslexia constitute evidence against models of reading which have just a semantic pathway, plus a 'direct' pathway necessary for nonword reading.

### (c) Lexical non-semantic reading

The classic case of this pattern of acquired dyslexia is WLP (Schwartz, Marin and Saffran, 1979; Schwartz, Saffran and Marin, 1980). This woman was suffering from a progressive dementing illness which in particular gravely affected her semantic abilities, whilst sparing syntax and phonology. When tested in March 1976, she performed at chance on the following semantic tests: (a) matching one of four pictures to a spoken word; (b) matching one of four pictures to a printed word; (c) categorising low-frequency nouns as animal versus body-part versus colour versus something else.

These results, plus her performance in picture-naming (very high error rate with profuse semantic errors), demonstrate the presence of a profound semantic impairment. This contrasted remarkably with her ability to read aloud – here she was fluent and accurate. Now, if there existed only the semantic and the non-lexical routes for reading, it would be possible for fluent and accurate reading to coexist with a semantic impairment only if the items being read were ones which could be read via the non-lexical route, that is, regular words and nonwords. Fluent and accurate reading of exception words would not be possible. Yet it was possible for WLP. In March 1976, she was given 22 exception words to read aloud; she read 21 of them correctly. Almost flawless reading aloud of exception words in the absence of an ability to comprehend

---

[1] We interpret his single success with pseudohomophonic nonwords, a correct reading of STAWK, as orthographically mediated, since his typical response to a nonword was a visually similar word.

written words is very difficult to explain except by postulating the existence of a lexical non-semantic reading route.

Two more recent cases (case DRN: Cipolotti and Warrington, 1995; case LAY: Cipolotti, 1995) provide similarly strong evidence for the existence of this third reading route. Both patients showed a serious single-word comprehension difficulty, particularly for low-frequency words. Comprehension was tested by asking the patients to define the words. Although their errors sometimes consisted of superordinate responses that indicate partial comprehension, the majority of their errors were either 'Don't know' responses, or were frankly erroneous. Both types of error indicate no access to any correct semantic information.

Reading aloud was, however, virtually perfect for both patients, and this included the reading aloud of low-frequency exception words.

Plaut et al. (1995), commenting on two of these three patients, say 'On our account, these observations suggest that, in these individuals, the phonological pathway had developed a relatively high degree of competence without assistance from semantics; but this post-hoc interpretation clearly requires some future, independent source of evidence'.

As discussed above, Plaut et al. (1995) proposed that the less literate a person is, the better the phonological pathway will be at reading exception words; that proposal allowed them to account for the severity difference between MP and KT in a non-ad-hoc way. Since WLP and the two Cipolotti patients were not even mild surface dyslexics despite their profound semantic impairments, on the PMSP interpretation their phonological pathways must have been essentially perfect at reading exception words. If so, all three must have been of very low premorbid literacy, even lower than MP. This prediction is not unreasonable re WLP, who was educated to the eighth grade and since then had been a mother, housewife and seamstress. But it is completely wrong for LAY, who had been a teacher, and even further off for DRN, who had been a biological scientist. Both of these people must have been highly literate premorbidly. The PMSP model thus predicts that a semantic impairment would make both patients profoundly surface dyslexic; but neither was surface dyslexic at all.

### (d) Conclusions regarding the PMSP simulations of acquired dyslexia

Simulating surface dyslexia has proven very difficult for this model and for the related SM model. The most natural move to make was to try to find a way to lesion the direct (phonological) route in a way that would harm exception words more than regular words and nonwords, and would produce regularisation errors in response to exception words. All efforts to do this failed. Hence attempts were made to simulate surface dyslexia as a lesion of the indirect (semantic) route, despite the inconvenience caused by the fact that this route is not implemented in the model. Provided the assumption is made that there is an inverse relationship between degree of literacy and the ability of the direct route to read exception words, the model could quantitatively simulate the data from the surface dyslexics MP and KT. But this assumption predicts that any person who was considerably or highly literate and has a severe semantic impairment will also be severely surface dyslexic, a prediction which is disconfirmed by the results of the studies of Cipolotti and Warrington (1995) and Cipolotti (1995). Thus the PMSP model's simulation of surface dyslexia is unsuccessful: it works only on the basis of an assumption which the empirical evidence refutes. We have also argued that the model's simulation of phonological dyslexia as involving reading via semantics is inconsistent with the results re WB reported by Funnell (1983); and that the model cannot simulate the pattern of acquired dyslexia known as lexical non-semantic reading because any explanation of this pattern requires the postulation of a third route from print to speech. Thus the data from all three forms of acquired dyslexia provide a most severe challenge to the PMSP model.

## Acquired dyslexias and the DRC model

### (a) Surface dyslexia

In terms of the traditional dual-route model, surface dyslexia occurs because of some impairment of the lexical route for reading. As discussed by Coltheart and Funnell (1987), there are several loci within such models where damage would produce the symptoms of surface dyslexia. The damage must be after the letter level (otherwise nonword reading would be affected too); and it must be before the phoneme level (for the same reason), but there remain several possible loci. In particular, damage to the phonological output lexicon would produce regularisation errors in reading exception words aloud, and at least one surface dyslexic appears to have this locus of damage (Kay and Ellis, 1987). However, other surface dyslexics such as HG (Coltheart and Funnell, 1987) and EE (Coltheart and Byng, 1989) appear to have an earlier deficit at or near the level of the orthographic input lexicon. Hence our initial work on simulating surface dyslexia focused on lesioning this region of the model.

As indicated earlier, with appropriate choice of parameters the DRC model correctly reads aloud all regular words, exception words and nonwords, and so would score 100% for all the kinds of stimuli represented in Figures 1.3 and 1.4. Our aim was to alter just a single parameter of the model, a parameter associated with the orthographic input lexicon, so as to leave the model's accuracy with regular words and nonwords intact, whilst causing it to make regularisation errors with exception words, and to make more such errors with low-frequency than with high-frequency exception words. The parameter we have studied so far is the one controlling the strength of the excitatory connections from letters to words. The value of this parameter is normally +0.070; that is, a set of parameters that allows the model to read regular words, nonwords and exception words perfectly has this value for letter-to-word excitation.

Reducing this value will reduce the rate at which activation grows in word units – that is, will impair the operation of the orthographic input lexicon – whilst leaving the operation of the other components of the model essentially unaffected.

Figure 1.5 shows the model's success in reading regular words, nonwords and exception words when the value of this parameter is reduced from +0.070 to +0.017. For comparison, the data from the surface dyslexic patient MP are included. Clearly, altering just a single parameter has changed the model from a normal reader to a surface dyslexic with levels of accuracy very similar to those shown by MP. All the errors made by the lesioned model were regularisation errors.

KT was more severely surface dyslexic than MP, so the relevant parameter must be reduced still further. Figure 1.6 shows the performance of the DRC model with letter-to-word activation reduced from its normal value of +0.070 to a value of +0.015. This yields an extremely close match between

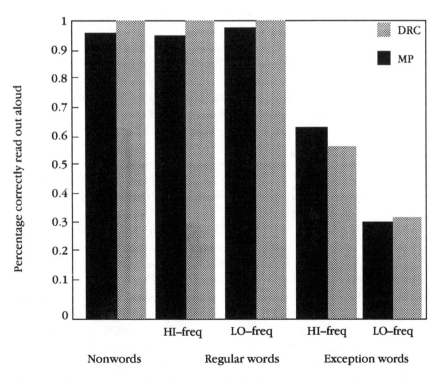

**Figure 1.5** Simulation of surface dyslexia. DRC model lesioned by reducing the strength of letter-to-word excitation from +0.07 to +0.017.

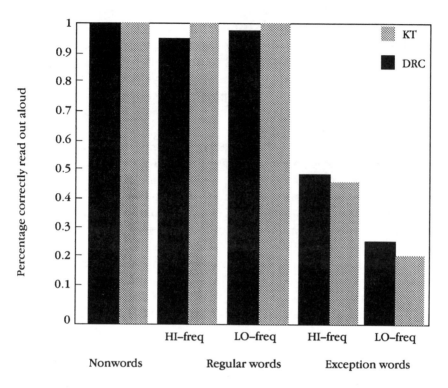

**Figure 1.6** Simulation of surface dyslexia. DRC model lesioned by reducing the strength of letter-to-word excitation from +0.07 to +0.015.

the lesioned model's reading accuracies and those of KT. Once again, all the errors made by the lesioned model were regularisation errors.

### (b) Phonological dyslexia

It is of course trivially easy for the DRC model to simulate severe phonological dyslexia – intact word reading with abolished nonword reading – by adjustment of just one parameter. Starting with a set of parameters that produce normal reading, the parameter controlling activation from the GPC route is reduced from its normal value to zero. Now all words are still read correctly by the model, but no nonword is.

More challenging is to attempt to simulate milder cases of phonological dyslexia. Figure 1.7 shows data from Derouesne and Beauvois (1985). Nonword reading by their patient LB was affected by two properties of nonwords, pseudohomophony and orthographic similarity. He read pseudohomophones better than nonpseudohomophones, and this effect was larger for pseudohomophones that are close to their parent word (an English example would be SAYL) than for those which are orthographically distant from their parent (an English example would be

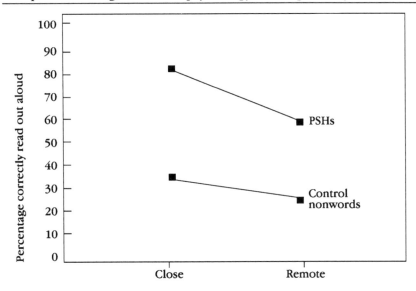

**Figure 1.7** Phonological dyslexia: patient LB. (PSHs: pseudohomophones.)

PHOCKS). Overall, LB read about 50% of nonwords correctly.

Thus we needed to discover whether one could lesion the DRC model in a way that would impair but not completely abolish nonword reading, and whether, if this could be done, the lesioned model's nonword reading would be sensitive to pseudohomophony and to orthographic similarity in the way the LB's reading was.

The one parameter we have worked with so far is that which controls the rate at which the GPC system delivers phonemes to the phoneme system. Because this system applies rules left to right, the first phoneme is delivered earlier than the second, and the second earlier than the third, and so on. The interval between successive phonemes in the set of parameters that yields normal reading (including perfect reading of all nonwords) is 7 processing cycles. That is, if the GPC route begins to deliver activation re the first phoneme to the phoneme level after X processing cycles, it begins to deliver activation re the second phoneme after X+7 cycles, the third after X+14 cycles, and so on.

When this value of 7 cycles is increased to 17 cycles, the DRC model's nonword reading accuracy drops from 100% to 33%, whilst its word reading accuracy remains at 100%. As Figure 1.8 shows, the reading of nonwords by this lesioned model is better for pseudohomophones than for nonpseudohomophones, and the pseudohomophone advantage is larger for pseudohomophones that are close to their parent word than for those which are not. Hence both of the effects seen in LB's nonword reading are also seen in the nonword reading of the lesioned DRC model. The simulation is certainly not perfect, because the absolute level of accuracy is lower in the model than in the patient, but what is important is that changing just a single parameter of

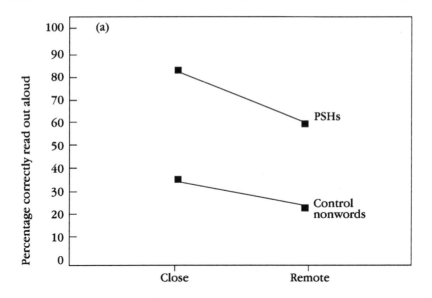

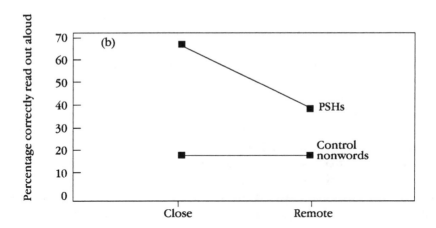

**Figure 1.8** Impaired nonword reading in phonological dyslexia: pseudohomo-phone advantage and its modulation by orthographic closeness to source word. (a) Patient LB. (b) Lesioned DRC model.

the model not only reduced nonword reading accuracy (it was obvious that this would happen) but introduced effects of pseudohomophony and orthographic similarity (it was not at all obvious that this would happen).

What is it about the DRC model that is responsible for the emergence of these two effects? Pseudohomophones are more resistant to the effects of lesioning the GPC route for the reason proposed by Derouesne and Beauvois (1985), namely, that activation at the phoneme level is supported interactively by the existence of a lexical entry in the phonological output lexicon for nonwords which are pseudohomophones. The orthographic proximity effect arises because nonword letter strings that are orthographically very close to real words partially excite the entries for these words in the orthographic input lexicon. In general, the majority of the phonemes in the pronunciation of any such word will also be in the pronunciation of the orthographically similar nonword. Therefore partial activation of the phoneme level arising from the partial activation at the level of the orthographic input lexicon will assist the reading of nonwords which are orthographically close to real words.

### (c) Lexical non-semantic reading

In its current form, DRC does not use a semantic system in its reading, so it reads exception words by lexical non-semantic reading. When a semantic route is implemented, this lexical non-semantic pathway will still be there. So simulation of lexical non-semantic reading poses no difficulties.

### (d) Conclusions regarding the DRC simulations of acquired dyslexia

Evidently, the DRC model is much more capable of simulating patterns of acquired dyslexia than is the PMSP model. One begins with a set of parameters which yield perfect reading of regular words, nonwords and exception words (and which successfully simulate various results from normal studies of lexical decision, reading aloud and priming). One then chooses just a single, theoretically relevant, parameter (in the case of surface dyslexia, letter-to-word excitation; in the case of phonological dyslexia, the rate of operation of the GPC route) and reduces it from its normal value, seeking a value which fits the patient data. Very close fits to data from two surface dyslexics, and a reasonable fit to data from one phonological dyslexic, have been obtained in this initial work; and clearly there are no difficulties regarding the simulation of lexical semantic reading.

## Conclusions

The theme of this book, 'Evaluating Theories of Language', could hardly be better illustrated than by the topic of this chapter, which is the application of data from patients with impaired reading to the task of constructing an adequate theory of how people normally recognise printed words and read them aloud. Our conclusion is that the cognitive neuropsychology of reading has, over the past two decades, yielded a multitude of results which would seem to demand that, whatever the detailed structure of the normal reading system is, the general architecture of this system must be modular, with distinct phonological and orthographic lexicons (directly connected to each other), a semantic system (connected to each of the two lexicons), and a separate system of non-lexical rules specifying correspondences between orthographic and phonological segments. No theory of reading that does not have that general architecture can be reconciled with what we now know about acquired dyslexias.

The next step forward is to seek to learn something about how these modules actually carry out their information-processing activities – which means to make the cognitive psychology of reading a computational cognitive psychology of reading, and to make the cognitive neuropsychology of reading a computational cognitive neuropsychology of reading. We have described two computational models of reading, and their application to the understanding of acquired dyslexias; and we have argued that data from studies of acquired reading impairment are especially illuminating here. These data are extremely difficult to reconcile with one of the models – and are very easily explained by the other.

# References

Baayen, R.H., Piepenbrock, R. and van Rijn, H. (1993). The CELEX Lexical Database (CD-ROM). Linguistic Data Consortium, University of Pennsylvania, Philadelphia, PA.

Besner, D., Twilley, L., McCann, R.S., & Seergobin, K. (1990). On the association between connectionism and data: Are a few words necessary? *Psychological Review*, 97, 432–446.

Bub, D., Cancelliere, A. and Kertesz, A. (1985). Whole-word and analytic translation of spelling-to-sound in a non-semantic reader. In K. Patterson, J.C. Marshall and M. Coltheart (Eds) *Surface Dyslexia: Neuropsychological and Cognitive Studies of Phonological Reading*, pp 15-34. London: Lawrence Erlbaum Associates.

Bullinaria, J.A. (1996). Representation, learning, generalization and damage in neural network models of reading aloud. Ms submitted for publication.

Cipolotti, L. (1995). British Psychological Society meeting, Warwick, UK, April.

Cipolotti, L. and Warrington, E.K. (1995). Semantic memory and reading abilities: A case report. *Neurocase*, 1, 104-110.

Coltheart, M. (1978). Lexical access in simple reading tasks. In G. Underwood (Ed.) *Strategies of Information Processing*. London: Academic Press.

Coltheart, M. (1985). Cognitive neurosychology and the study of reading. In Posner, M.I and O.S.M. Marin (eds), Attention and Performance XI (p. 3–37). Hillsdale, NJ: Erlbaum.

Coltheart, M. (1994). Connectionist modelling and cognitive psychology. *Noetica* 1 (1).

Coltheart, M. (1995). Simulation of acquired dyslexia by the DRC model, a computational model of visual word recognition, reading aloud and spelling. Presented at the conference on Neural Modelling of Cognitive and Brain Disorders, University of Maryland, 8-10 June.

Coltheart, M. and Byng, S. (1989). A treatment for surface dyslexia. In X. Seron (Ed.)

*Cognitive Approaches in Neuropsychological Rehabilitation*. London: Lawrence Erlbaum Associates.

Coltheart, M. and Funnell, E. (1987). Reading and writing: one lexicon or two? In D.A. Allport, D.G. MacKay, W. Prinz and E. Scheerer (Eds) *Language Perception and Production: Shared Mechanisms in Listening, Reading and Writing*. London: Academic Press.

Coltheart, M. and Rastle, K. (1994). A left-to-right serial process in reading aloud. Journal of Experimental Psychology: *Human Perception and Performance*, **20**, 1197-1211.

Coltheart, M., Curtis, B. Atkins, P. and Haller, M. (1993). Models of reading aloud: Dual-route and parallel-distributed-processing approaches. *Psychological Review*, **100**, 589-608.

Derouesne, J. and Beauvois, M-F. (1985). The 'phonemic' stage in the non-lexical reading process: Evidence from a case of phonological alexia. In K. Patterson, J.C. Marshall and M. Coltheart (Eds) *Surface Dyslexia: Neuropsychological and Cognitive Studies of Phonological Reading*, pp. 399-457. London: Lawrence Erlbaum Associates.

Ellis, A.W. and Young, A.W. (1988). *Human Cognitive Neuropsychology*. London: Lawrence Erlbaum Associates.

Funnell, E. (1983). Phonological processer in reading: Evidence from acquired dyslexia. *British Journal of Psychology*, **74**, 159–180.

Kay, J. and Ellis, A.W (1987). A cognitive neuropsychological case study of anomia: Implications for psychological models of word retrieval. *Brain*, **110**, 613-629.

Marshall, J.C. and Newcombe, F. (1973). Patterns of paralexia: A psycholinguistic approach. *Journal of Psycholinguistic Research*, **2**, 175-199.

McCarthy, R. and Warrington, E.K. (1986). Phonological reading: Phenomena and paradoxes. *Cortex*, **22**, 359-380.

McCarthy, R. and Warrington, E.K. (1990). *Cognitive Neuropsychology: a Clinical Introduction*. San Diego: Academic Press.

Mozer, M. and Behrmann, M.P. (1990). On the interaction of selective attention and lexical knowledge: A connectionist account of neglect dyslexia. *Journal of Cognitive Neuroscience*, **2**, 96-123.

Paap, K.R. and Noel, R.W. (1991). Dual route models of print to sound: Still a good horse race. *Psychological Research*, **53**, 13-24.

Patel, M. and Coltheart, M. (1996). Work in progress.

Patterson, K. (1990). Alexia and neural nets. *Japanese Journal of Psychology*, **6**, 90-99.

Patterson, K. and Shewell, C. (1987). Speak and spell: dissociations and word-class effects. In M. Coltheart, G. Sartori, and R. Job (Eds) *The Cognitive Neuropsychology of Language*. London: Lawrence Erlbaum Associates.

Patterson, K., Seidenberg, M.S. and McClelland, J.L. (1989). Connections and disconnections: Acquired dyslexia in a computational model of reading processes. In R.G.M. Morris (Ed.) *Parallel Distributed Processing: Implications for Psychology and Neuroscience*, pp. 131-181. London: Oxford University Press.

Plaut, D.C. and Shallice, T. (1993). Deep dyslexia: A case study of connectionist neuropsychology. *Cognitive Neuropsychology*, **10**, 377-500.

Plaut, D.C., McClelland, J.L., Seidenberg, M.S. and Patterson, K. (1995). Understanding normal and impaired word reading: Computational principles in quasi-regular domains. *Psychological Review*, in press.

Reggia, J.A., Marsland, P.M. and Berndt, R.S. (1988). Competitive dynamics in a dual-route connectionist model of print-to-sound transformation. *Complex Systems*, **2**, 509-547.

Saffran, E.M. (1982). Neuropsychological approaches to the study of language. *British Journal of Psychology*, **73**, 317-337.

Schwartz, M.F., Marin, O.S.M. and Saffran, E. (1979). Dissociations of language function in dementia: A case study. *Brain and Language*, **7**, 277-306.

Schwartz, M.F., Saffran, E. and Marin, O.S.M. (1980). Fractionating the reading process in dementia: Evidence for word-specific print-to-sound associations. In M. Coltheart, K. Patterson and J.C. Marshall (Eds) *Deep Dyslexia*. London: Routledge and Kegan Paul.

Seidenberg, M.S. (1988). Cognitive neuropsychology and language: The state of the art. *Cognitive Neuropsychology*, **5**, 403-426.

Seidenberg, M.S. and McClelland, J.L. (1989). A distributed, developmental model of word recognition and naming. *Psychological Review*, **69**, 523-568.

Seidenberg, M., Waters, G.S., Barnes, M.A. and Tanenhaus, M. (1984). When does irregular spelling or pronunciation influence word recognition? *Journal of Verbal Learning and Verbal Behaviour*, **23**, 383-404.

Shallice, T. (1988). *From Neuropsychology to Mental Structure*. Cambridge: Cambridge University Press.

Shallice, T., Warrington E.K. and McCarthy, R. (1983). Reading without semantics. *Quarterly Journal of Experimental Psychology*, **35A**, 111-138.

Taraban, R. and McClelland, J.L. (1987). conspiracy effects in word pronunciation. *Journal of Memory and Language*, **26**, 608-631.

Zorzi, M., Houghton, G. and Butterworth, B. (1995). Two routes or one in reading aloud? A connectionist dual- route model. *Technical Report*, UCL.RRG.95.1, University College London.

# Chapter 2
# From Snarks to Boojums: Why Are Prosodic Disabilities So Rare?

PAUL. F. McCORMACK

They sought it with thimbles, they sought it with care;
They pursued it with forks and hope;
They threatened its life with a railway-share;
They charmed it with smiles and soap.
They hunted till darkness came on, but they found
Not a button, or feather, or mark,
By which they could tell that they stood on the ground
Where the Baker had met with the Snark.
In the midst of the word he was trying to say,
In the midst of his laughter and glee,
He had softly and suddenly vanished away -
For the Snark **was** a Boojum, you see.
from *The Hunting of the Snark* by Lewis Carroll (1876)

## Abstract

*Disturbances to prosody are often reported in cases of neurologically acquired speech and language disorders. What is not clear is the extent to which such disturbances reflect a disruption to prosodic organisation itself, and, if it is affected, what aspects of that organisation are involved. Research to date is notably ambiguous as to whether primary disturbances to prosody actually occur compared with those that arise as secondary consequences to disruptions at other levels of linguistic or non-linguistic functioning. The evidence is far from convincing that discrete areas of the brain are responsible for particular aspects of prosodic functioning. Nor is there convincing evidence of cases where a prosodic disturbance at the phonological level (a prosodic disability) has been identified in contrast to one at the phonetic level (a dysprosody). It will be argued that clearly identified phonological based prosodic disturbances are rare (if they occur at all) because the functions and organisation of prosodic phonology are fundamentally different from those of segmental phonology. Prosody is neither autonomous from other levels of linguistic organisation, nor is its main linguistic function to code paradigmatic phonological contrasts. Prosody's main role, while linguistic, is organisational, and its contrastive functioning is syntagmatic. Thus a number of current assessment procedures for prosody that are based on testing quasi-paradigmatic contrasts do not appropriately reflect its functioning and organisation. The challenge for researchers is to develop appropriate descriptive and experimental frameworks that are based more closely on the way prosody functions in communication.*

## Introduction

One of the 'wildcards' in the study of speech and language is prosody. It still remains one of the least understood and least agreed upon areas in phonetics and linguistics (Beckman, 1995). This uncertainty about prosody is perhaps even greater in neurolinguistics where points of view are more varied than found amongst linguists and phoneticians (Ryalls, 1986; Lesser, 1989). Snark-hunting may only be for the foolhardy, and it may be wiser to leave such unpredictable beasts as prosody and prosodic disorder well alone, but, as bravely as the Baker, I want to suggest that an exploration of some of the reasons that underlie this lack of development compared with other areas of speech and language behaviour could prove very fruitful in the pursuit of this book's theme: the limits to which disordered speech and language can inform us about the processes involved in normal communication.

The questions I wish to explore are not so much why and how prosodic disabilities arise, but why they do not occur more than they do? Why, when they do occur, are they usually so limited in nature? And finally, what does the *absence* of a speech disorder tell us about the organisation of speech and language? I hope to convince the reader that the reason why prosodic disabilities are so rare is the same reason why so little progress has been made in achieving a widely agreed framework for the definition and description of prosody. The phonological organisation of prosody is essentially different from that found with speech segments themselves. As a result, its functions in the process of communication are markedly different from segmental phonology.

Segmental phonology is usually defined and described as an autonomous component of speech and language organisation (Lass, 1984). Its contrastive role in the expression of meaning is dependent on this autonomy from other levels of linguistic organisation. Thus it is only indirectly constrained by semantics, syntax and morphology. Traditionally, linguists have viewed segmental phonology as a low level but key component in the communication of meaning, whereby a small set of arbitrary speech sounds combine to produce higher level grammatical units. This 'double articulation' of language provides its potential for infinite flexibility (Lyons, 1986). Such a self-contained system is vulnerable to significant internal disruption when placed under demand (Shattuck-Hufnagel, 1986; Levelt, 1989).

Prosody, while recognised by linguists as a distinct phonological system involved in the expression of meaning, does not function independently from other levels of speech and language organisation. Its phonological units are directly constrained by semantic, syntactic and morphological factors (Couper-Kuhlen, 1986). Prosody is also highly sensitive to and reflective of such extralinguistic factors as a person's emotional state (Bolinger, 1985). It is this direct dependence that accounts for the perennial difficulty in defining and describing the limits of prosody. It also accounts for its vulnerability to external disruption, where changes in prosody arise as secondary consequences to primary disturbances at other levels of linguistic organisation (Ryalls, 1986; Brewster, 1989).

This direct dependence of prosody on other levels of language organisation also provides one of the main reasons for its extraordinary robustness as a phonological system in the presence of neurological impairment. Prosodic disabilities are rare because prosody, while distinct, is not organised as an autonomous and discrete linguistic system. Concomitantly, one cannot expect the neurological substrates of prosodic organisation to reflect anything but this high level of dependency on this wide and diverse range of language and speech domains. This was a point made by Monrad-Krohn nearly 50 years ago in his seminal work on prosodic disturbances that arise from neurological impairment:

> I have no intention of trying to localise this 'prosodic faculty' to those numerous shades of meaning which this prosodic faculty alone can convey, co-operation of the whole brain is probably needed. (Monrad-Krohn, 1947: 415).

There is also another reason why prosody is so resistant to a primary disturbance at the phonological level. It has become increasingly recognised by phoneticians, linguists and psycholinguists that one of the main phonological functions of prosody is the provision of the organisational framework for the spoken message (Selkirk, 1984; Beckman, 1986; Nespor and Vogel, 1986; Levelt, 1989). Shattuck-Hufnagel's (1986) 'slots and fillers' theory of speech production provides a vivid model of this relationship at the phonological level between prosody and speech segments: prior to the establishment of the segmental phonological plan a prosodic template of an utterance is generated which provides the framework (slots) into which speech segments (fillers) are slotted. Normal speech errors ('slips of the tongue') overwhelmingly involve transpositions of speech segments that are highly constrained by the prosodic structure of the utterance.

# Prosodic disorders

The discussion of prosody and disorders of prosody in neurolinguistics is bedevilled by confusions arising from vagueness in the use of terminology and considerable variation in the aspect of prosody being investigated (Ryalls, 1986; Lesser, 1989). For example, Darley, Aronson and Brown (1975) describe prosody as '...all the variations in time, pitch, and loudness that accomplish emphasis, lend interest to speech, and characterise individual and dialectal modes of expression' (p. 5). Code (1987) treats prosody as a non-linguistic aspect of speech with no propositional role in communication. Ross (1981) develops a complete classification system for 'aprosodias' based on affective criteria alone, while Cooper and Zurif (1983) consider prosody only in terms of being a direct suprasegmental expression of syntactic constraints. Other researchers have taken a more linguistic approach to prosody in as much as they have investigated aspects of prosody that have been traditionally seen as providing semantic contrasts in English. Examples of these more linguistically focused approaches to prosody would be investigations of the perception or production of rising versus falling pitch contours as expressions of interrogatives versus statements, or investigations of differences between compound nouns and noun phrases (Blumstein and Goodglass, 1972; Behrens, 1987; Darkins, Fromkin and Benson, 1988).

The question of disturbed prosody has been a common theme in the study of the linguistic effects of brain impairment since Chacot (1877). Monrad-Krohn (1947) has provided the most influential model for classifying neurologically based prosodic disturbances. Most prosodic disorders were described as either 'aprosodic' (lacking any prosodic expression), 'hyperprosodic' (increased prosodic expression) or 'dysprosodic' (disordered prosodic expression). Monrad-Krohn associated the first two prosodic disturbances with problems associated with muscle control, while the third he considered might possibly arise from a disturbance to prosodic functioning itself. Such a disturbance arose from 'higher up' in the central nervous system than those associated with muscle control. The classic examples provided by Monrad-Krohn are the prosodic disturbance that arises from damage to the cerebellum (ataxic dysarthria), and that arising from a case of cortical damage that led to the perception of a 'foreign accent'. Certainly the impression given by Monrad-Krohn that most prosodic disturbances arise from neurological impairments in muscle movements (dysarthria) seems borne out by the distribution of reports in the literature. The overwhelming number of studies commenting on prosody in neurological damage relate to the dysarthrias (Kent, 1990). There are a substantial number of studies, however, that report on the prosodic characteristics that arise from neurological damage not primarily associated with dysarthria. These involve damage to both the left and right cortical hemispheres, and are associated with aphasias or verbal dyspraxias. Table 2.1 outlines the traditional three-tiered model of neurological speech disorders as outlined by McNeil and Kent (1990), and the type of speech disorder, be it segmental or prosodic, that can arise from impairment at a particular level of neurological organisation. However, the clear demarcation between the characteristics of neurological speech disorders and the assumption that the identified levels do not systematically interact is no longer tenable (McNeil and Kent, 1990; McCormack, 1995).

**Table 2.1** Traditional three-tiered model of neurological speech disorders (after McNeil and Kent, 1990)

| | | |
|---|---|---|
| Aphasia | > | Phonological plan |
| Verbal apraxia | > | Phonetic (motor programming) |
| Dysarthria | > | Articulatory (motor execution) |

Researchers on the dysarthrias have traditionally been concerned with describing and understanding speech patterns beyond the domain of individual speech segments and words. They have long recognised that segmentally focused descriptions were not appropriate. However, the way they have approached prosodic phenomena has involved simplifying the complexity of prosody by focusing on only discrete phonetic exponents such as 'loudness' or 'average pitch and range of pitch movement'. Any role that prosody might have in linguistic organisation and functioning is usually ignored. This results in piecemeal investigations of quite limited aspects of prosody. For example, in the classic perceptual studies of the dysarthrias by Darley, Aronson and Brown (1975) prosody was confusingly treated as being part of a number of dimensions rated by judges. One was 'phonatory–prosodic insufficiency'. The indications of such insufficiency were monopitch, monoloudness and harsh voice quality. As the name of this dimension implies, it focuses on perceptual characteristics arising from changes in laryngeal functioning. Another dimension was 'prosodic excess' which referred to the perception of 'phoneme prolongations', 'prolonged intervals', 'monoloudness', and 'excess and equal stress'. Essentially such an approach to some features of prosodic behaviour is phonetic in focus, but the selection of these behaviours is completely arbitrary and without any theoretical justification or perspective. Different aspects of some phonetic exponents of prosody such as pitch movement, loudness and duration are mixed with articulatory and laryngeal factors. More recently such perceptual investigations of prosody in dysarthria have been complemented by acoustic or articulatory-instrumental studies (Hertrich and Ackermann, 1993; Hirose, 1986). Such studies are still limited to descriptively investigating discrete components described as 'prosodic', but without reference to how such components relate to prosody as a whole and function in speech organisation. In this sense they are not really studies of prosody, nor are they truly phonetic, since even the most basic phonetic descriptions are based on some theory of how speech is organised. Because these studies are so narrowly focused on measuring physiological 'outputs' with little reference to the possible significance as to whether the 'input' is linguistic or not, they often have little to contribute to the understanding of any prosodic disturbance except in rather crude reductionist terms (Weismer and Liss, 1991).

## The notion of 'prosodic disability'

Initially, one may be puzzled by the assertion that acquired prosodic disabilities are rare. The literature is replete with studies of disturbed prosody in cases of dysarthria (Darley, Aronson and Brown, 1975; Kent and Rosenbek, 1982; McCormack and Ingram, 1995), dyspraxia (Blumstein, 1973; Kean, 1977), aphasia (Blumstein, 1973, 1995), 'foreign accent syndrome' (Blumstein, Alexander, Ryalls, Katz and Dworetsky, 1987; Ingram, McCormack and Kennedy, 1992), and right hemisphere damage (Code, 1987; Oellette and Baum, 1993). An informal review of the research studies published in the last five years in *Brain and Language* or *The Journal of Speech and Hearing Research* indicated that in studies investigating some aspect of speech, over 30% made some reference to disturbances in the perception or production of prosody. However, I am restricting the use of the term *prosodic disability* to the sense that Crystal (1981, 1984) and Brewster (1989) have proposed. A prosodic disability refers to a primary disturbance to the linguistic organisation of prosody itself, rather than as arising as either a secondary consequence of a disturbance in some other aspect of linguistic or non-linguistic organisation, or as a problem with the phonetic control of a prosodic feature such as pitch or timing. Crystal (1981) defines a prosodic disorder that arises from a low-level motor impairment (i.e. phonetic) as a *dysprosody*, while one that arises as a consequence of a problem at another level of linguistic organisation (such as syntax or semantics) is described as a *prosodic disturbance*.

Crystal's work has been a major force in opening up the field of neurolinguistics to basic linguistic theory. The classification system proposed by Crystal (1981) is linguistically motivated and parallels the types of distinctions made in the study of segmental speech both in linguistics and neurolinguistics (Blumstein, 1995). The critical feature of this approach is the notion that one can distinguish between the phonological and the phonetic levels of description. This distinction between phonological and phonetic levels in the organisation of speech has been the driving force behind the development of modern phonology (Jakobson and Waugh, 1979). So too in neurolinguistics, this distinction has provided the fundamental framework for the interpretation of segmental speech errors arising from neurological impairments (Blumstein, 1973; Crystal, 1984; Lesser, 1989). For example, it is a commonly held view that some forms of aphasia result in phonological speech errors in addition to any errors that may arise due to problems with phonetic implementation (Kean, 1995). I wish to argue that, unlike the evidence for phonological disturbances in segmental speech errors (Blumstein, 1973; Kean, 1995), there is no evidence (or at least no unambiguous evidence) that primary disturbances in the phonological organisation of prosody occur subsequent to neurological damage. As well as being a general observation made from surveying published studies, it is also by way of a critique of two hypotheses proposed by Crystal (1981, 1982, 1984). The first is that prosodic disabilities are analogous in their form to segmental speech disabilities, and result in the form of reduced prosodic systems. I want to argue that such loss of the system of prosodic contrasts rarely if ever occurs. The only researcher who seems to have reported such a form of phonological disability is Crystal himself (1981, 1982, 1984), and these reports are fragmentary in their description. Crystal's hypothesis about the nature of prosodic disabilities, which provides the rationale for his clinical descriptive procedure the PROP (Prosody Profile, 1982), is founded more on a deductively based theory of prosodic organisation rather than on clear inductive evidence. The second hypothesis by Crystal (1981, 1982, 1984) is that the majority of prosodic disabilities involve the intonational system (the system of pitch contrasts). Again, this is a somewhat unique view of how prosodic disturbances mainly manifest themselves, and appears to be founded more on theoretical assumptions about prosodic organisation rather than on a strong base of empirical evidence. Crystal (1969) holds the strong opinion that some aspects of prosody are more 'linguistic' than others, with the intonation system being the most linguistic. This is his main justification for the PROP being essentially an analysis of intonation. I want to propose a contrary viewpoint; that most reported prosodic disturbances affecting the ability to communicate effectively have predominantly involved changes in speech timing and phrasing (Kent and Rosenbek, 1982; Gandour, 1987; Moen, 1991; Kent, 1990). Disturbances in the perception and production of linguistic stress and rhythm are much more common than Crystal's model of prosodic disorders gives credit (Kent, 1990).

At issue here is the difficulty in distinguishing between the phonological and phonetic levels of representation for prosody. A range of criteria based on categorical distinctions in meaning can be utilised with speech segments to determine their phonological status (Lass, 1984) (for example, using a minimal pair 'test' such as 'fish'/'dish'). This has been a powerful heuristic device for studying segmental speech errors in neurolinguistics (Blumstein, 1995; Kean, 1995). However, the expression of meaning by prosodic means arises predominantly through gradient changes rather than as the result of specific categorical contrasts (Bolinger, 1985). To 'test' the phonological status of particular aspects of prosody using criteria that reflect principles of segmental speech organisation may be inappropriate and misrepresent their actual functioning in the language. For example, it has been common in neurolinguistics to examine the phonological status of prosodic disturbances by utilising quasi-paradigmatically focused material such as noun/verb contrasts (e.g. *IMport versus imPORT*), compound noun/noun phrase contrasts (*a WETsuit* versus *a wetSUIT*), or differences in syntactic status attributed to rising or falling intonation patterns (Behrens, 1987; Darkins, Fromkin and Benson, 1988; Bryan, 1989; Peppe, Bryan and Maxim, 1995). Yet I would suggest that these are aspects of the functioning of prosody that are either quite peripheral or have misinterpreted its phonological role. If this is indeed the case, then such assessment material will not provide a satisfactory means of assessing the neurolinguistic status of prosodic disturbances. Current research results with this type of material, while sometimes indicating increased numbers of prosodic errors, have not demonstrated the existence of qualitatively changed prosodic systems. To understand these differences of opinion about what might constitute a phonological problem with prosody, it would be worthwhile to review briefly how linguists have come to think about prosody this century.

## Twentieth century approaches to prosody

A clear phonological role for prosody has only strongly and consistently emerged in the mainstream phonological literature over the last three decades (Chomsky and Halle, 1968; Liberman and Prince, 1977; Selkirk, 1984; Goldsmith, 1990). This role has emerged as phonological theories have begun to consider that the organisational characteristics of speech as a complex sequence of sounds are, at least in part, linguistically determined, and thus part of a speaker's language competence. Previously phonologists tended to focus predominantly on establishing individual phonological units in terms of their distinctiveness or paradigmatic contrastiveness with each other (Bloomfield, 1933). Thus in English /p/ potentially (paradigmatically) contrasts with /b/ and with /m/ in such words as *pat*, *bat* and *mat*. Non-contrastive aspects of speech tended to be viewed as redundant and non-linguistic, and therefore outside the domain of phonology proper. Prosodic constructs that had no perceivable contrastive function such as syllable structure, stress feet, and rhythm belonged to the domain of universal principles of perceptual or motor performance, and were thus, at best, phonetic. A contrastive function for prosody was perceived as very limited, being restricted to some aspects of intonation and word-stress (Saussure, 1916; Bloomfield,

1933; Crystal, 1969). For example, in English there are a handful of quasi-paradigmatic contrasts such as the rising and falling pitch patterns commonly associated with interrogatives versus statements, or the stress contrasts for word pairs such as *REcord* (noun) versus *reCORD* (verb), or the stress contrasts for some compound noun forms with particular noun phrases such as *HOTdog* (compound noun) versus *hot DOG* (noun phrase).

However, such an approach to prosody cannot adequately account for the pattern of stresses in English. Word-stress contrasts of this type form only a minuscule percentage of the word-stress patterns found in English. In the majority of English words the distribution of stresses do not result in critical contrasts of lexical meaning and do not serve such a linguistic function. More importantly, unlike the tones in tone languages, the stress contrasts that do occur are not directly derived from paradigmatic substitutions. Rather the contrasts are syntagmatic (sequential), arising from the position of the stress within the whole syllable pattern of the word. Referring to the above example, in *REcord* the first syllable carries the primary stress, while in *reCORD* it is the second syllable. The contrast arises not from changes in one particular segment or syllable per se, but from the relative prominence pattern in the whole word. Qualities of the other syllable also contribute to the overall perception of the prominence pattern for that word (Beckman, 1986). Further to this, as phonetic studies of stress have indicated, there is no simple and direct phonetic quality from which any 'stress contrast' could be derived (Gimson, 1980; Pittam and Ingram, 1992). The paradigmatic approach to stress is both phonologically and phonetically unrealistic, yet it often forms the basis for testing the linguistic status of a prosodic disorder. For such approaches to analysing prosody see Crystal's PROP (1982), Darkins et al. (1988), Bryan (1989), and Peppe, Bryan and Maxim (1995).

In contrast to this rather restricted view of prosody, there have also been proponents of a more general linguistic (phonological) function for prosody in terms of its organising role (Trubetzkoy, 1939; Bolinger, 1961; Jakobson and Waugh, 1979). In the 1920s, 30s, and 40s phonologists in the Prague Linguistic Circle proposed that phonology should not be viewed as solely concerned with paradigmatic contrasts. There were two types of function subserved by phonological patterns. Firstly there were paradigmatic sound patterns, and secondly, there were syntagmatic sound patterns. Paradigmatic relationships between sound segments were such that particular segments within a language's speech sound system were in potential contrast with each other. A sound segment was a phonological unit if it produced a distinctive contrast in meaning when it substituted for other speech segments. However, there were also syntagmatic relationships between sound units which Trubetzkoy (1939) termed 'configurative'. These reflected the relationships found in the combination of sound units and which extended beyond individual segments as such, giving unity and organisation to the sound pattern. Syntagmatic relationships involved speech sounds that were present within the same utterance, or stretch of utterance. This gave an utterance a configurative unity based on the positions of prominent elements in its organisation. Both Trubetzkoy (1939) and Jakobson (Jakobson and Waugh, 1979) viewed the configurative syntagmatic function in phonology as very important, but secondary to the distinctive paradigmatic function.

This recognition that the relationships between elements in an utterance were part of the phonology of a language provided an effective foil to the 'phonological-means-phonemic' school of thought. The work of the Prague Circle on exploring the wider range of phonological functions in language has been highly influential in motivating phonologists to consider prosodic phenomena as a central part of linguistics rather than a peripheral concern (Lass, 1984). In this notion of 'configurative features' one can see the forerunner of such contemporary notions as 'stress contour' (Chomsky and Halle, 1968), 'phonological phrasing' (Nespor and Vogel, 1986), 'metrical constituency' (Liberman and Prince, 1977; Selkirk, 1984), and 'prosodic grouping' (Hirst, 1993). The basic assumption underlying such terminology is that phonological units join together to form larger units which have their own principles of organisation. To assess the linguistic status of a prosodic disorder should involve investigating its critical role in organising the configurative unity of what is said.

There has been one other influential approach to prosody that has much in common with the approach of the Prague Circle. British phoneticians and phonologists have traditionally focused on both the organisational and contrastive aspects of prosodic patterning. Their descriptions have emphasised the organisation of prosody into units spanning the utterance or parts of the utterance. The basic units were defined as tone units and stress groups (feet). These units have hierarchical internal structures, which, in the case of intonation, have elaborate specifications (Crystal, 1969; Gimson, 1980). These sub-constituents of the tone unit are truly syntagmatic in their relationship with the other sub-constituents. Each is dependent for their definition on their position in relation to the other sub-constituents. For example, by definition, the pre-head precedes the head, the head precedes the nucleus, and the tail follows the nucleus. At the same time as the development of these detailed phonetic descriptions of the syntagmatic organisation of prosodic units, British scholars were also elaborating the range of meanings expressed by different aspects of prosodic organisation. In a sense these were paradigmatic contrasts, in as much as they reflected closed sets of prosodic features that could occur in a particular part of the tone unit. The sense of contrast was different than that found in segmental phonology, however, since there was a recognition of gradations in the prosodic expression of meaning rather than the system of discrete categorical meaning contrasts found amongst speech segments (Crystal, 1969). An example of this quasi-paradigmatic approach to interpreting prosodic function is the detailed analysis by O'Connor and Arnold (1973) of the intonational 'tunes' of English as expressing dozens of discrete types of meaning. Each tune is paradigmatically distinctive in as much as each expresses a different meaning and is potentially contrastive with other possible tunes within the system. The exact meaning of the tune, however, is dependent on the characteristics of the tune over the whole utterance, and gradations of meaning could be associated with subtle nuances in the expression of those tunes. The difficulty has been that such elaborate systems of contrast have proved to be unreliable and have been rejected by most linguists. More recently, it has been suggested that these nuances of meaning could be viewed as sharing one contrastive role of expressing the speaker's 'commitment' (high tone) or 'lack of commitment' (low tone) to aspects of a discourse (Pierrehumbert and Hirschberg, 1990).

Crystal (1969, 1981, 1982) provides an example of the continuation of this direct phonetic approach to defining prosodic phenomena. In *Prosodic Systems and Intonation in English*, Crystal (1969) outlines an elaborate taxonomy of prosodic systems, with each system based on a distinct phonetic parameter. The intonation system is based on pitch movements, the stress system is based on variations in loudness, rhythm is based on the durations between syllables, the pause system is based on the position and duration of pauses, and the tempo system is based on the durations within syllables. To justify this elaborate range of distinct systems, however, Crystal (1969) is forced into the paradoxical position of supporting phonetic criteria of dubious empirical validity. Although acknowledging and discussing the research indicating that pitch rather than loudness was a more effective cue to stress, Crystal maintains a model of prosody and prosodic disorders where stress is described as having the dominant perceptual basis of loudness. Crystal (1969, 1975, 1981, 1982) also displays the dichotomy about prosody that is found generally in the British approach. On the one hand there is the explicit phonetic model of prosodic features based on their syntagmatic organisation. On the other hand, the phonological functions of those syntagmatic characteristics are ignored at the expense of emphasising quasi-paradigmatic contrastiveness. It seems that only 'contrastiveness' is linguistic:

> Some non-segmental features have a very high degree of internal patterning and contrastivity, similar to the segmental contrasts and duality implicit in the rest of language; others are substantially less discrete in their definition and less systemic in their

function, being much closer to the range of completely non-
linguistic vocal effects...At the 'most linguistic' extreme would be
placed those prosodic features of utterance, describable in terms
of closed systems of contrasts, which are relatively easily integrated with other aspects of linguistic structure, particularly
grammar, ... At the other, 'least linguistic' end would be placed
those paralinguistic features of an utterance which seem to have
little potential for entering into systemic relationships. (Crystal,
1969: 129)

Crystal (1969) proposes a clearly demarcated framework for considering prosodic speech characteristics as being either 'linguistic' or 'non-
linguistic'. This same perspective underlies his approach to prosodic
disorders (Crystal, 1981, 1982, 1984). He argues that there are degrees
of 'grammaticality' in prosody. Intonation was the most 'phonological'
system. The stress system is less grammatical than the intonation system
because many stress placements, either at the lexical level or in
connected speech do not alter the meaning of the message. Speech
rhythm was the least grammatical of the major prosodic systems because
of its high degree of unpredictable variation. This variation is of importance for all prosodic phenomena. Bolinger (1961, 1985) has noted that
'gradience', the expression of a phonological characteristic by degrees
rather than in an 'all-or-nothing' categorical way, is a feature of all
prosodic behaviour. The issue is whether because a parameter is gradient in its expression it is therefore not 'linguistic' in its functioning. At
the segmental level of speech organisation the criterion of categorical
distinctiveness has been regarded as a touchstone for determining the
phonological level of organisation from the purely phonetic. Many studies of speech changes in acquired neurological speech disorders have
relied on this criterion for determining whether a speech disorder was
phonological or phonetic (Brewster, 1989; Blumstein, 1990). The fact
that prosody is mainly gradient in its expression, however, has meant
that studies of prosodic disorders have been hampered by the difficulty
in establishing the criteria for determining what level of speech organisation is involved. This has tended to restrict empirical investigations of
prosodic disorders either to descriptive studies of prosodic output (Kent
and Rosenbek, 1982; Hertrich and Ackerman, 1993), or, as argued
above, to testing quasi-paradigmatic prosodic contrasts which margin-
alise the main functions of prosody by focusing on peripheral phenomena (Behrens, 1987; Darkins et al., 1988; Bryan, 1989; Peppe et al.,
1995).
    As indicated by a succession of authors, attempts to localise discrete
prosodic functions to particular areas of the brain have been essentially
flawed by their assumptions about the nature of prosody and its relationships to other levels of linguistic organisation (Monrad-Krohn, 1947;

Ryalls, 1986; Moen, 1991; Oellette and Baum, 1993). The discrete quasi-paradigmatic contrasts utilised in a number of assessments of prosodic disorders do not appropriately reflect prosody's functioning and organisation as reflected in current linguistic, phonetic and psycholinguistic thought. The challenge for researchers is to develop appropriate descriptive and experimental frameworks that are based more closely on the way prosody functions in communication.

## Conclusion

There is a lesson to be learned from this non-conformist behaviour of prosody and prosodic disorders. Bolinger (1985) used the story of Cinderella as a metaphor for the state of neglect that the study of prosody has been in compared with other aspects of speech and language organisation. Lesser (1989) used the same metaphor to describe a parallel state of neglect for prosodic disorders in neurolinguistics. Perhaps the time has come to extend the metaphor a little further. By the end of the story Cinderella moves from an insignificant position to one at the centre of affairs. So too with prosody there has been growth in the perception of the role of prosody in the organisation and functioning of speech and language. This has arisen out of the increasing perception by a number of different disciplines that the main role of prosody has never been contrastiveness but rather as the organising principle of speech. Rather than viewing prosody as only marginally linguistic (Bloomfield, 1933; Crystal, 1969) contemporary phonologies increasingly place non-segmental aspects of speech such as syllable structure and metrical and intonational organisation at the heart of how speech is represented phonologically (Goldsmith, 1990). In phonetics, the syntagmatic organisation of speaking has traditionally been viewed as important for understanding how individual speech sounds are realised (Gimson, 1980). More recently the evidence for the fundamental role of prosody in this process has been increasing as phonetics has begun to be more concerned with modelling the characteristics of connected speech (Kohler, 1995). In psycholinguistics a number of contemporary models of speech production, for example the 'slots and fillers' model (Shattuk-Hufnagel, 1986), Levelt's (1989), and Ferreira's (1993) models rely heavily on the premise that prosody provides the pivotal structure around which speech planning is organised.

The evidence is not so clear for prosodic disorders taking a more central role in the development of neurolinguistics. Some of this may be due to 'lag time' between shifts in perspective in linguistics and psycholinguistics and their subsequent informing of neurolinguistic research. However, much is no doubt due to the general confusion that still hangs over the definition of prosody and prosodic disturbances in the neurolinguistic literature, as well as uncertainty about how prosody can be evaluated appropriately in subjects with neurological impairment. Nevertheless there are trends emerging from a number of independent researchers that seem to indicate that there is a fundamental dichotomy in the way that the brain perceives and produces the timing characteristics of speech compared with that of fundamental frequency. While Crystal (1981) had proposed that the main forms of prosodic disability involved intonational errors (its acoustic correlate being movement in fundamental frequency), many researchers have found that disturbances in the control of speech timing are much more pervasive and critical for functioning in cortical and subcortical damage (Blumstein and Cooper, 1974; Danly, Cooper and Shapiro, 1983; Gandour, 1987; Moen, 1991; Hertrich and Ackermann, 1993; McCormack, 1995). But even so, there is little if any evidence of any primary phonological impairment.

I want to leave the last word to Lewis Carroll again. He has the wise advice that to hunt Snarks you need the right type of map, and perhaps no map is better than using the wrong one. However, the second to last word is left to Sheila Blumstein (1995) whose pioneering work on speech errors has shaped much of the current perspective on neurolinguistics. At the XIIIth Congress of Phonetic Sciences in Stockholm she proposed that the speech errors that arise from neurological impairment reflect difficulties with processing rather than impairments to linguistic or phonetic organisation itself. If prosody's principle function involves the provision of the organisational structure for speech, and its contrastiveness is syntagmatic rather than paradigmatic, then it becomes even clearer why the phonological representation of prosody is rarely if ever disturbed.

> The pattern of both speech production and speech perception deficits in aphasia suggest that the disorders reflect impairments to the processes involved in accessing the sound structure rather than selective impairments to the sound properties of speech or to their representations. Speech production deficits occur at both the phonological level, reflecting selection or access impairments, as well as at the phonetic level, reflecting articulatory implementation impairments.(Blumstein, 1995: 180).

So how successful have we been in hunting Snarks? Have we any clearer notions about the nature and role of prosody from this absence (or at least dearth) of prosodic disabilities? I think we do. The main lesson is that we must put away the conventional maps of the relationship between phonology and phonetics if we are to investigate prosodic disorders and their relationship to normal prosodic function. While the traditional notion of paradigmatic contrastiveness may assist us with understanding the segmental organisation of speech and disorders that can arise with neurological damage, such a notion will continue to mislead us in the pursuit of prosody and its disturbance. And as Blumstein (1995) indicates above, even the types of segmental speech errors arising from neurological impairment are more than likely less straight-forward than traditionally conceived.

> He had bought a large map representing the sea,
> Without the least vestige of land:
> And the crew were much pleased when they found it to be
> A map they could all understand.

> What's the good of Mercator's North Poles and Equators,
> Tropics, Zones, and Meridian Lines?'
> So the Bellman would cry: and the crew would reply,
> 'They are merely conventional signs!'

> 'Other maps are such shapes, with their islands and capes!
> But we've got our brave Captain to thank'
> (So the crew would protest) 'that he's bought us the best -
> A perfect and absolute blank!"
> from *The Hunting of the Snark* by Lewis Carroll (1876)

# References

Baum, S., Daniloff, J., Daniloff, R. and Lewis, J. (1982). Sentence comprehension by Broca's aphasics: Effects of some suprasegmental variables. *Brain and Language*, 17, 261–271.

Beckman, M. (1986). *Stress and Non-Stress Accent*. Dordrecht: Foris.

Beckman, M. (1995). Problems of intonation. In G. Bloothooft, V. Hazan, D. Huber, and J. Llisterri (Eds) *European Studies in Phonetics and Speech Communication*, pp. 148–158. Utrecht: OTS Publications.

Behrens, S. (1987). The role of the right hemisphere in the production of linguistic prosody: An acoustic investigation. In J. Ryalls (Ed.) *Phonetic Approaches to Speech Production in Aphasia and Related Disorders*, pp. 81–92, Boston: College-Hill.

Bloomfield, L. (1933). *Language*. New York: Holt, Rinehart & Winston.

Blumstein, S. (1973). *A Phonological Investigation of Aphasic Speech*. The Hague: Mouton.

Blumstein, S. (1990). Phonological deficits in aphasia: Theoretical perspectives. In A. Caramazza (Ed.) *Cognitive Neuropsychology and Neurolinguistics: Advances in Models of Cognitive Function and Impairment*, pp. 33–53. New Jersey: Lawrence Erlbaum.

Blumstein, S. (1995). On the neurobiology of the sound structure of language: Evidence from aphasia. In K. Elenius and P. Branderud (Eds) *Proceedings of The XIIIth International Congress of Phonetic Sciences*, Volume 2, pp. 180–185. Stockholm: KTH and Stockholm Universities.

Blumstein, S. and Cooper, W. (1974). Hemispheric processing of intonation contours. *Cortex*, 10, 146–158.

Blumstein, S. and Goodglass, H. (1972). The perception of stress as a semantic cue in aphasia. *Journal of Speech and Hearing Research*, 15, 800–806.

Blumstein, S., Alexander, M., Ryalls, J., Katz, W. and Dworetsky, B. (1987). On the nature of foreign accent syndrome: a case-study. *Brain and Language*, 31, 215–244.

Bolinger, D. (1961). *Generality, Gradience, and the All-or-none*. The Hague: Mouton.

Bolinger, D. (1985). *Intonation and its parts: Melody in spoken English*. London: Edward Arnold.

Brewster, K. (1989). Assessment of prosody. In K. Grundy (Ed.) *Linguistics in Clinical Practice*, pp. 168–185. London: Taylor & Francis.

Bryan, K. (1989). Language prosody and the right hemisphere. *Aphasiology*, 3, 285–299.

Chacot J. (1877). *Lectures on the Diseases of the Nervous System*. London: New Sydenham Society.

Chomsky, N. and Halle, M. (1968). *The Sound Pattern of English*. New York: Harper & Row.

Code, C. (1987). *Language, Aphasia, and the Right Hemisphere*. Chichester: John Wiley & Sons.

Cooper, W. and Zurif, E. (1983). Aphasia: Information-processing in language production and reception. In B. Butterworth (Ed.) *Language Production*, Vol. 2, pp. 225–249. London: Academic Press.

Couper-Kuhlen, E. (1986). *An Introduction to English Prosody*. London: Edward Arnold.

Crystal, D. (1969). *Prosodic Systems and Intonation in English*. Cambridge: Cambridge University Press.

Crystal, D. (1981). *Clinical Linguistics*. Vienna: Springer.

Crystal, D. (1982). *Profiling Linguistic Disability*. London: Edward Arnold.

Crystal, D. (1984). *Linguistic Encounters with Language Handicap*. Oxford: Blackwell.

Danly, M., Cooper, W. and Shapiro, B. (1983). Fundamental frequency, language processing, and linguistic structure in Wernicke's aphasia. *Brain and Language*, 19, 1–24.

Darkins, A., Fromkin, V. and Benson, D. (1988). A characterization of the prosodic loss in Parkinson's disease. *Brain and Language*, 34, 315–327.

Darley, F., Aronson, A. and Brown, J. (1975). *Motor Speech Disorders*. Philadelphia: Saunders.

Emmorey, K. (1987). The neurological substrates of prosodic aspects of speech. *Brain and Language*, 30, 305–320.

Ferreira, F. (1993). The creation of prosody during sentence production. *Psychological Review*, 50, 233–253.

Gandour, J. (1987). Tone production in aphasia. In J. Ryalls (Ed.) *Phonetic Approaches to Speech Production in Aphasia and Related Disorders*, pp. 45–57. Boston: College-Hill Press.

Gardener, M. (1962). *The Annotated Snark*. Harmondsworth: Penguin Books.

Gimson, A. (1980). *An Introduction to the Pronunciation of English*, 3rd edition. London: Edward Arnold.

Goldsmith, J. (1990). *Autosegmental and Metrical Phonology*. Oxford: Blackwell.

Goodglass, H., Fodor, I. and Schulhoff, C. (1967). Prosodic factors in grammar – evidence from aphasia. *Journal of Speech and Hearing Research*, 10, 5–20.

Hertrich, I. and Ackermann, H. (1993). Acoustic analysis of speech prosody in Huntington's and Parkinson's disease: a preliminary report. *Clinical Linguistics and Phonetics*, 7 (4), 285–297.

Hirose, H. (1986). Pathophysiology of motor speech disorders (dysarthria). *Folia Phoniatrica*, 38, 61–88.

Hirst, D. (1993). Peak, boundary and cohesion characteristics of prosodic grouping, in D. House and P. Touati (Eds) *Working Papers* 41, pp. 32–37. Sweden: Lund University Department of Linguistics.

Ingram, J., McCormack, P. and Kennedy, M. (1992). The phonetic analysis of a case of foreign accent syndrome. *Journal of Phonetics*, **20** (4), 457–474.

Jakobson, R. and Waugh, L. (1979). *The Sound Shape of Language*. Sussex: The Harvester Press.

Kean, M. (1977). The linguistic interpretation of aphasic syndromes: agrammatism in Broca's aphasia, an example. *Cognition*, **5**, 9–46.

Kean, M. (1995). Phonological structure and the analysis of phonemic paraphasias. In K. Elenius and P. Branderud (Eds) *Proceedings of The XIIIth International Congress of Phonetic Sciences*, Volume 2, pp. 186–192. Stockholm: KTH and Stockholm Universities.

Kent, R.D. (1990). The acoustic and physiologic characteristics of neurologically impaired speech movements. In W.J. Hardcastle and A. Marchal (Eds) *Speech Production and Speech Modelling*, pp. 365–402. Dordrecht: Kluwer Academic Pub.

Kent, R. and Rosenbek, J. (1982). Prosodic disturbance and neurologic lesion. *Brain and Language*, **15**, 259–291.

Kohler, K. (1995). Phonetics and Speech Communication: Past Development and Future Perspectives. In G. Bloothooft, V. Hazan, D. Huber, and J. Llisterri (Eds) *European Studies in Phonetics and Speech Communication*, pp. 18–22. Utrecht: OTS Publications.

Lass, R. (1984) *Phonology*. Cambridge: Cambridge University Press.

Lesser, R. (1989). *Linguistic Investigations of Aphasia*, Second Edition. London: Cole & Whurr.

Levelt, W. (1989). *Speaking: From Intention to Articulation*. Cambridge, Mass.: MIT Press.

Liberman, M. and Prince, A. (1977). On stress and linguistic rhythm. *Linguistic Inquiry*, **8**, 249–336.

Lyons, J. (1986) *Language and Linguistics*. Cambridge: Cambridge University Press.

McCormack, P. (1995). *The Rhythm Rule in Normal and Ataxic Speech Production*. Unpublished doctoral dissertation. University of Queensland.

McCormack, P. and Ingram, J. (1995). Anticipatory motor programming in ataxic dysarthria. In K. Elenius and P. Branderud (Eds) *Proceedings of The XIIIth International Congress of Phonetic Sciences.*, Volume 4, pp. 512–515. Stockholm: KTH and Stockholm Universities.

McNeil, M. and Kent, R. (1990). Motoric characteristics of adult aphasic and apraxic speakers. In G. Hammond (Ed.) *Cerebral Control of Speech and Limb Movements*, pp. 349–386. Amsterdam: Elsevier/North Holland.

Moen, I. (1991). Functional lateralisation of pitch accents and intonation in Norwegian: Monrad-Krohn's study of an aphasic patient with altered 'melody of speech'. *Brain and Language*, **41** (4), 538–554.

Monrad-Krohn, G. (1947). Dysprosody or altered 'melody of language'. *Brain*, **70**, 405–415.

Nespor, M. and Vogel, I. (1986). *Prosodic Phonology*. Dordrecht: Foris.

O'Connor, J. and Arnold, G. (1973). *The Intonation of Colloquial English*, 2nd edition. London: Longman.

Oellette, G. and Baum, S. (1993). Acoustic analysis of prosodic cues in left- and right-hemisphere-damaged patients. *Aphasiology*, **8** (3), 257–283.

Peppe, S., Bryan, K. and Maxim J. (1995). Prosody in aphasia: An assessment procedure and 3 case-studies. In M. Kersner and S. Peppe (Eds) *Work in Progress*, Volume 5. Department of Human Communication Science, University College London.

Pierrehumbert, J. and Hirschberg, J. (1990). The meaning of intonation contours in the interpretation of discourse. In P. Cohen, J. Morgan and M. Pollack (Eds) *Intentions in Communication*, pp. 271–311. Cambridge MA: MIT.

Pittam, J. and Ingram, J. (1992). Accuracy of perception and production of compound and phrasal stress by Vietnamese-Australians. *Applied Psycholinguistics*, **13**(1), 1–12.

Ross, E. (1981). The aprosodias: Functional-anatomical organization of the affective components of language in the right hemisphere. *Archives of Neurology*, **38**, 561–569.

Ryalls, J. (1986). What constitutes a primary disturbance of speech prosody? *Brain and Language*, **29**, 183–187.

Saussure, F. de (1916). *Cours de linguistique generale*. Paris: Payot.

Selkirk, E. (1984). *Phonology and Syntax: The Relationship Between Sound and Structure*. Cambridge, Mass.: MIT Press.

Shattuk-Hufnagel, S. (1986). The representation of phonological information during speech production planning: Evidence from vowel errors in spontaneous speech. *Phonology Yearbook*, **3**, 117–149.

Trubetzkoy, N. (1939). *Principles of Phonology*. English edition (1969) translated by C. Baltaxe. Los Angeles: University of California Press.

Weismer, G. and Liss, J. (1991). Reductionism is a dead-end in speech research. In C. Moore, K. Yrokston and D. Deukelman (Eds) *Dysarthria and Apraxia of Speech: Perspectives on Management*, pp. 15–27. Baltimore: Paul H. Brookes.

# Chapter 3
# Underlying Representations in the Acquisition of Phonology: Evidence from 'Before and After' Speech

ANDREW BUTCHER

## Abstract

*An issue which has been central to the modelling of the acquisition of phonology over the years – going back at least to Smith (1973) and Waterson (1971) – is the question of how many levels of underlying representation are postulated. Do we have (at least during the acquisition stage) a lexicon of forms used in perception and a separate lexicon of forms for production, or do we have a single common lexicon which underlies both aspects of the speech process? Two-lexicon models claim to account better for a number of commonly observed phenomena such as lexical avoidance, context-conditioning of 'rules', and variability of phonetic output. This chapter discusses the implications for this debate of some data (partly anecdotal, partly quantitative) on the 'late acquisition' of some key phonological contrasts. At least one current version of the 'two-lexicon' model (Hewlett, 1990) envisages the acquisition of forms in the output lexicon as proceeding via a gradual development and automatisation of motor programmes based on forms from the input lexicon. Results of work with postoperative cleft palate speakers, and with a child with glue ear after grommet insertion, show a rapidity of acquisition of appropriate and consistent pronunciations for coronal fricatives and voicing of initial stops respectively which appears to be incompatible with the notion of gradual development of a separate output lexicon.*

## Introduction

The speech behaviour of individuals with less than perfect mastery of the normal adult system is often regarded as a 'window' offering potential illumination of the extremely complex and largely opaque processes of speech perception and production. One of the most obvious of such windows, and one which has received much attention from linguists over the last few decades is that offered by the child acquiring language. One of the central issues in the modelling of speech processing has been the nature and number of abstract levels of representation that are postulated. Since language acquisition proceeds in stages, there is some reason to suppose that the corresponding changes in the form of the child's words may reflect changes at different levels of representation. Thus a study of the nature of such changes may provide the linguist with some insight into the nature of the underlying representations.

In 1973, Neil Smith published his seminal account of the acquisition of English phonology by his son (Smith, 1973). In this and in subsequent papers (e.g. Smith, 1981) he argued that children possess a capacity for speech perception which is more or less equivalent to that of an adult and that the phonology thus has a single abstract underlying representation in the child's brain which is from an early stage effectively the same as the adult's. The well attested and much described differences between the speech of an adult and the speech of a child acquiring language are thus, according to Smith's generative phonology approach, fully interpretable in terms of phonetic realisation rules operating on individual phonemes. The child's non-adult pronunciations are seen as solely attributable to immaturity in the ability to exercise control over various aspects of the speech production process, in particular supra-laryngeal articulation and its coordination with laryngeal gestures.

Over this same period of time, Natalie Waterson was approaching the issue from the perspective of prosodic phonology (Waterson, 1971, 1981). She argued that the child does not initially perceive in an adult way, and that therefore the underlying representation is not equivalent to the adult's. In fact, according to Waterson's model, there are two levels of underlying representation, and the child initially does not resemble the adult at either level. Underlying representation number one (URI), on the input side of the process, is a store of possible phonetic patterns of the language, with no associated meanings, used in 'speech reception and recognition'. For Waterson it is the output lexicon which appears to be more central to the speech process. Underlying representation number two (URII) is a store of 'lexical-phonological patterns', with associated meanings and full phonetic specification, which is 'concerned with interpretation and production' (Waterson, 1981: 326f). URII is constructed on the basis of URI. Perceptual processing is a matter of matching patterns between URI and URII. Waterson suggests four stages in the acquisition process. In the initial stage both underlying representations and the child's articulatory abilities are unlike the adult's. At the second stage URI, the input lexicon, has become adult-like, but URII, the output lexicon, has not. At stage three both underlying representations now resemble those of the adult, but the child's pronunciation may still differ because of production constraints. At the final stage, URI, URII and the production ability all match those of the adult.

The cognitive psychological approach represented by Menn, Ferguson, Macken and others also shows a preference for (though not a reliance on) the postulation of two levels of representation. Menn (1983: 9) claims that:

> To advocate a single lexicon ... is to hypothesize that the rules which create the child's output form from her input form operate in real time; to advocate a two-lexicon model is to claim that a form 'closer' to the output form is also stored and that this second form is used as a basis for production.

Menn also adopts Waterson's notion of the canonical form, as 'a program in which some parameters are fixed, but others are settable'. Such a programme (or rather, programme specification) is one step up from the completely invariant 'phonological idiom', where all parameters are fixed. The learning of canonical forms represents an automatisation of part of the speech production process. Entries in the output lexicon now consist of a canonical form plus a value for each variable parameter. The production of a word entails recalling the appropriate form plus the parameter values from the output lexicon and then 'plugging in' the values into the articulatory programme specified by the canonical form. Phonological development consists of increasing the number of parameters which can be varied within a canonical form, increasing the range of variation of each parameter, and concatenating short forms, or 'programmes', to make longer ones.

One of the most recent versions of the 'two-lexicon' model is that of Hewlett (1990), who also proposes one set of phonological representations which are perceptually based 'and therefore reflect phonological contrasts available to the child in decoding speech', and one set which are articulatorily based and 'reflect pronunciation abilities'. In normal speech development the input lexicon is richer in contrasts than the output lexicon, and the correspondences between these levels of representation are expressed through 'process'-type rules. Like Menn, he stresses the point that in a two-lexicon model such rules need not operate in real time. In contrast to his predecessors, Hewlett gives rather more detailed consideration to the role of motor programming, processing and execution. In his model it is the input lexicon which appears to be the more fundamental of the two: the motor programmer initially puts together the motor plan for the production of a given form on the basis of input it receives from the input lexicon. The motor processing component chooses the parameter values within the motor plan and

adjusts them on the basis of feedback from the motor execution component. This is 'the slow route'. Successful motor plans are used to
develop mapping rules between the input lexicon and the output lexicon. Thus the latter is little more than a set of stored programmes. As the
system becomes more practised in implementing a given plan, the
implementation is increasingly 'fast-tracked' by being delegated to the
motor processing component. Thus both Menn and Hewlett emphasise
that acquisition of adult-like production involves attainment of a high
degree of automaticity. Figure 3.1 shows the essential features of a
generic two-lexicon model of the speech process.

Hewlett's model specifically addresses a number of issues which had
previously remained somewhat unclear. One problem is the relationship
between the output lexicon and the constraints on production imposed

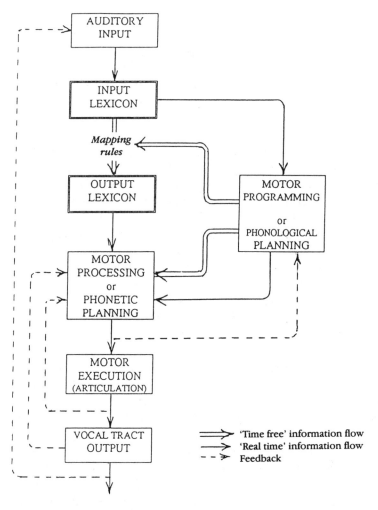

**Figure 3.1** Main features of a two-lexicon model of the speech process.

by the immature motor control of the vocal tract. Waterson, for example, at one stage (1981: 329) states that 'as URII [= the output lexicon] is constructed on the basis of URI [= the input lexicon], URII is considered to change before there is a change in production' – in other words underlying forms in the output lexicon determine what the pronunciation patterns will be. On the other hand, when discussing a specific example of changing pronunciation, she postulates a stage at which the child's 'URI pattern will have these [place of articulation] features, but production difficulties mean that his URII pattern will still differ from the adult's' (p. 330). At this point she seems to be saying that the child's actual pronunciation pattern determines what the form in the output lexicon will be. Menn is not clear on this point, but Hewlett (1990: 32) is quite unambiguous. He suggests that if adjustment of the parameter values within the motor plan by the motor processing component is not sufficient to produce a satisfactory output, the motor programmer may extend or modify the parameters of the plan or devise an entirely different plan, and thus alter the specification of the form in the output lexicon itself.

Not all current research in the area of normal and disordered phonological acquisition assumes a two-lexicon model. Dodd, Leahy and Hambly (1989), for example, discuss different speech patterns in different groups of speech disordered children in terms of a single mental lexicon. A very basic generic single-lexicon model is schematised in Figure 3.2. Clearly the main difference from the two-lexicon model, as Menn (1983) has pointed out, is that rules which map input forms to output forms apply between the single lexicon and the motor processing stage and therefore must operate in real time. There seem to be a couple of unwarranted assumptions about the nature of such models which are not, however, intrinsic to them. One assumption appears to be that a single-lexicon model implies that all output constraints must be explained in terms of low-level phonetic realisation rules. In other words, there is no provision for the automatisation of motor plans, unless these are to be 'phonologised' in a separate output lexicon. A second, related assumption is that there is no possibility within the single-lexicon model for the by-passing of automated output forms in order to account for better performance in imitation tasks than in spontaneous speech. Dodd et al. (1989) show that neither of these assumptions is implicit in the single lexicon model. Firstly differences between child and adult output are explained in terms of evolving hypotheses derived from the lexicon about the nature of the phonological system. These hypotheses are used to generate realisation rules which in turn constrain the output of a phonological planning component, which is responsible for the selection and sequencing of phonemes. Secondly there is provision for a direct link between the perceptual analysis of input surface forms and the planning component which completely by-passes both the lexicon and the realisation rules.

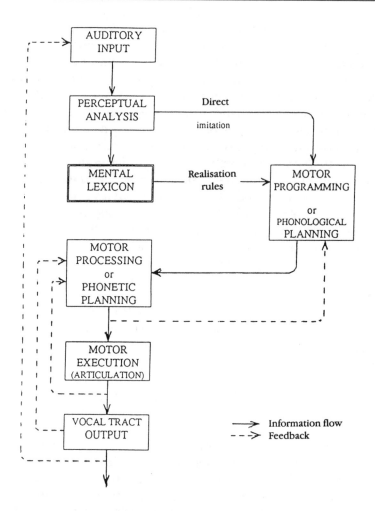

**Figure 3.2** Main features of a single-lexicon model of the speech process.

It is arguable that further light may be shed on these issues by studying the acquisition of phonology by speakers whose speech and/or language faculties are impaired. A number of studies have considered the question of underlying representations in the light of data from different groups of speakers diagnosed with different types of speech disorder, which have been compared with group data from normal subjects (e.g. Dodd et al., 1989; Williams and Chiat 1993). There are a number of limitations to this approach, however. The chief of these is that the nature of the impairment is rarely independently verifiable, but has to be inferred from the output. In a somewhat circular manner, conclusions are then drawn as to the effect of this type of impairment on the speech and language patterns of the subjects. A second problem is that group studies typically fail to take account of the wide degree of variation shown among normal speakers.

In this chapter I will pursue the less usual course of considering some individual cases of speech impairment. In these cases more adult-like speech output has been achieved by means of changes in known and specific 'independent variables' effected through surgical intervention. These changes were made at 'opposite ends' of the speech process – in the first two cases in the vocal tract itself and in the third case at the level of auditory input.

## The case of postoperative cleft palate speakers

This section briefly reviews some published data on cleft palate speakers who produced substitute sounds for coronal obstruents. In both cases, abnormal speech patterns were analysed and subsequently remediated using electropalatography (EPG). Full details of the system are given in Hardcastle, Gibbon and Jones (1991). Briefly, the technique requires the use of an electropalate – a denture-like acrylic plate (without teeth), which is individually moulded to fit the palate of each speaker. Mounted on the underside of this plate are 62 silver electrodes, each of which is connected to a thin copper wire. The wires emerge at the posterior corners of the plate and are led out at the corners of the mouth to plug into a multiplexer unit hung around the speaker's neck, which is in turn connected (via optical isolators) to the EPG control unit, and thence to the computer. During recording the speaker holds a hand electrode connected to the control unit, which supplies a very small AC signal to the body. This signal is conducted from the tongue to the palate electrodes whenever contact is made. The electrodes are scanned at a sampling rate of 100 Hz, i.e. once every 10 ms. The changing patterns of linguo-palatal contact may be displayed in real time on the computer screen, together with an intensity-related signal derived from the microphone input, and stored for subsequent reviewing, editing or printing out in the form of a series of 'electropalatograms'. In these diagrams the front of the electropalate (the immediate post-dental region) is at the top and the back (the border between hard and soft palates) is at the bottom. Electrodes in contact with the tongue are represented by filled circles; inactive electrodes are represented by open circles.

The case of PB is described by Dent, Gibbon and Hardcastle (1992) and Hardcastle, Gibbon and Dent (1994). He was born with a unilateral cleft lip and palate, had a lip repair at 3 months and a palate repair at 6 months, with further lip revision at 4;6. He had received regular speech therapy since 1;0. At 2;0 he had delayed speech and expressive language development, bilateral conductive hearing loss and a retracted (velar) place of articulation for many sound classes. By 4;0 his hearing was within normal limits, and at 4;6 his speech was described as containing variable velar substitutions, distortions and cluster reductions. At 9;6, with language skills by this time judged to be age appropriate, he was referred for EPG-based therapy. PB's main problem at this time was the abnormal production of /s/ and /z/, which were produced as nasopharyn-

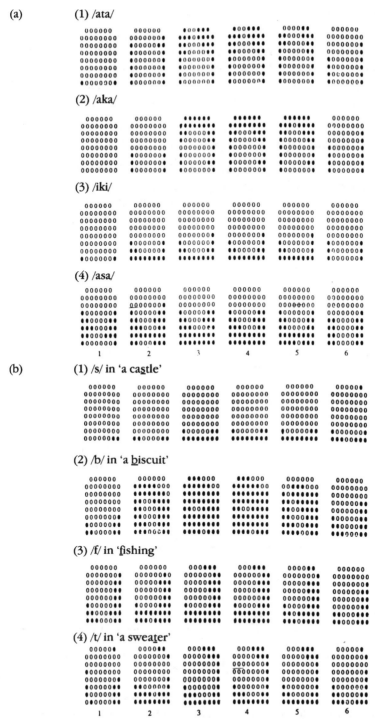

**Figure 3.3** EPG printout showing six stages in the articulation of (a) normal speaker's production of /t/, /s/ and /k/ and (b) PB's production of /s/ and /t/ prior to therapy (adapted from Dent et al., 1992: Figures 25.3 and 25.4).

geal fricatives. There was also complete velar contact for these and most other sounds, together with varying degrees of nasal emission. Figure 3.3 compares typical EPG patterns from PB's speech with those of a normal speaker. Importantly, Dent et al state (p. 216) that 'radiographic recordings suggested that P had adequate velopharyngeal competence. It was felt that the nasal emission could be due instead to an abnormal learned motor pattern ... rather than an inadequate mechanism'.

Therapy was aimed at modifying tongue behaviour to eradicate the inappropriate double articulations (which were thought also to contribute to the perception of increased nasality) and to establish the tongue tip rather than the tongue body as the articulator for alveolar fricative sounds. According to Hardcastle et al. (1994: 161), both of these objectives were achieved: 'after a few clinical sessions, PB was able to monitor his own production of these sounds and produce at will the anterior stop with and without accompanying velar closure'. As Figure 3.4 shows, alveolar articulations now show contact in the alveolar region (with some grooving for fricatives) and complete disappearance of the inappropriate velar contact and concomitant reduction of perceived nasality.

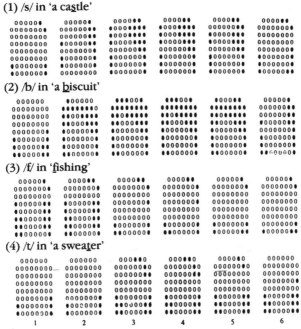

**Figure 3.4** EPG printout showing six stages in the articulation of PB's production of /s/ and /t/ following therapy (adapted from Dent et al., 1992: Figure 25.5).

The second case is that of TG, described by Hardcastle, Dent and Gibbon (1992) and Hardcastle, Gibbon and Dent (1994). This speaker was only diagnosed with velopharyngeal incompetence at 3;6, and a pharyngoplasty was not carried out until 6;1. He had a unilateral sensorineural–neural hearing loss, but age-appropriate language skills. By age 9;0, despite regular conventional speech therapy, TG was still producing all lingual obstruents with minimal tongue–palate contact. In particular /s/ and / ʃ / were apparently produced as pharyngeal fricatives (compare (a) and (b) of Figure 3.5). The aim of therapy was to develop a range of new motor patterns appropriate to the normal articulation of lingual fricatives and stops. As can be seen from the examples in Figure 3.5 (c), this aim was achieved. According to Hardcastle et al. (1994: 160) 'the newly learned patterns had obviously been mastered with dramatic improvement in overall intelligibility'.

(a)

(b)

(c)

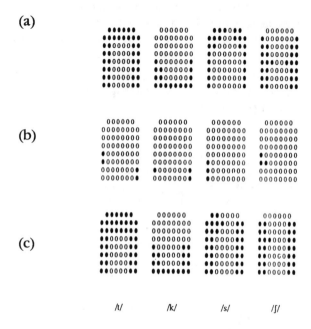

/t/             /k/             /s/             /ʃ/

**Figure 3.5** EPG patterns at point of maximum constriction for a number of lingual obstruent sounds as articulated by a normal speaker (a) and by TG before (b) and after (c) therapy (adapted from Hardcastle et al., 1994: Figures 5 and 6).

## A case of glue ear

The final case, which I will consider in somewhat more detail, is that of LS, a 6-year-old with normal receptive and expressive language skills, diagnosed as having a slight high-frequency conductive hearing loss. As well as a number of other minor phonological problems, he was unable to produce a contrast between voiced and voiceless stops in any position in the word. According to two commonly used criteria, this could be categorised as a phonological disorder. Firstly, the lack of contrast was quite consistent in LS's speech and secondly, and more importantly, it affected both prevocalic and postvocalic positions, involving quite different motor programmes. LS was recorded in a quiet room, using a good quality analogue cassette tape recorder and an external cardioid condenser microphone, as he carried out two tasks. In the first task he pronounced a number of monosyllabic words by naming a set of pictures. In the second he repeated these same words after the model of the speech therapist. The recordings were digitised to hard disk at a sampling rate of 20.05 kHz with 16-bit resolution. Acoustic measurements were carried out using the ESPS/waves+ signal processing software.

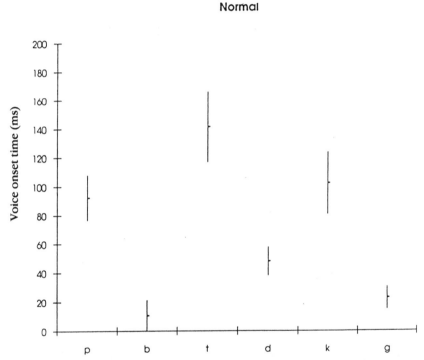

**Figure 3.6** Means and standard deviations of voice onset times for initial stops in the speech of a normal 6-year-old.

Figure 3.6 shows how a normal 6-year-old distinguishes initial stops in terms of voice onset time (VOT). Note that values for voiceless stops are on average over three times those for voiced stops. As Figure 3.7 clearly shows, LS failed to distinguish initial stops in monosyllables elicited by picture naming. Across all places of articulation there was no difference in VOT between voiced and voiceless targets, whereas VOTs for voiceless stops are over three times as long as those for voiced stops in the normal child. The problem was that all LS's initial stops sounded voiceless. His VOTs were all entirely appropriate to voiceless plosives, and he was apparently incapable of reducing VOT to a duration appropriate for the corresponding voiced sounds. Although his performance improved slightly under imitation conditions, VOTs for voiceless stops were, on average, still only 12 % longer than those for voiced ones, which is not a significant difference. Moreover, the difference between the overall VOT differences under the two conditions is also not significant (in all cases *p* < 0.05 by *t*-test for paired samples).

(a)

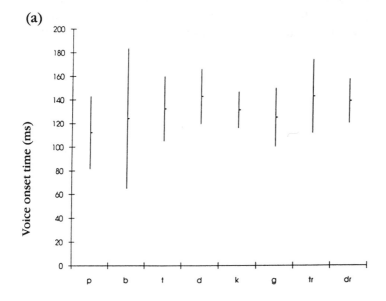

(b)

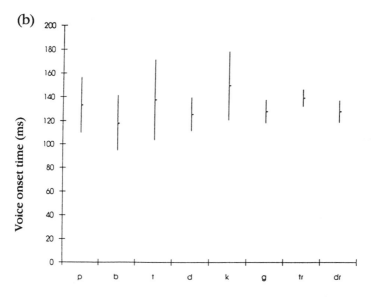

**Figure 3.7** Means and standard deviations of voice onset times for initial stops in the speech of LS before bilateral myringotomy and grommet insertion. (a) in elicitation task (b) in imitation task

Figure 3.8 shows that the problem with the voicing distinction in final position is much less severe – at least with regard to what is arguably the main acoustic cue: the duration of the preceding vowel. Long vowels and diphthongs in the speech of normal adults are about twice as long before final voiced obstruents as before final voiceless ones. Short vowels are in the order of 30% longer before voiced obstruents. In the case of LS's

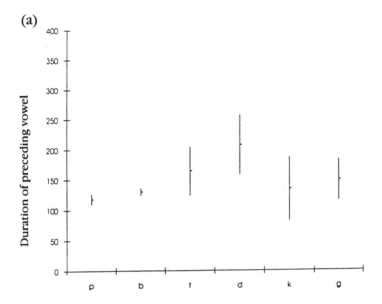

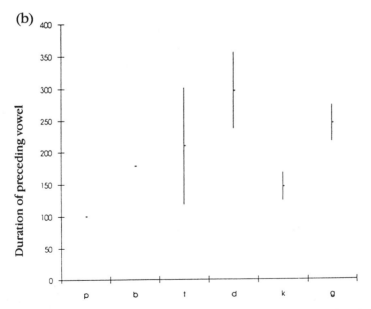

**Figure 3.8** Means and standard deviations of vowel durations before final stops in the speech of LS before bilateral myringotomy and grommet insertion. (a) in elicitation task (b) in imitation task

elicited speech there was an overall difference in mean duration which was statistically significant, but not consistently adequate. Vowels before voiced consonants were on average 19% longer than those before voice-less ones. In the imitated forms the differences approached normal adult proportions, with vowels before voiced consonants 54% longer, although standard deviations for /t/ and /d/ are very high and there is no significant difference between the elicitation and imitation conditions.

LS's problem was quite resistant to therapy and, at the insistence of his parents, a second opinion was sought regarding his hearing loss. The second otorhinolaryngologist diagnosed secretory otitis media and recommended bilateral myringotomy with grommet insertion, which was carried out shortly afterwards. Approximately one week after this operation he returned for speech therapy and showed dramatic improvements in his production of the voicing distinction. In particular, VOTs for initial voiced targets were now significantly reduced. A recording was made of him at this session, using the same list of words under the same conditions as before.

Figure 3.9 shows that VOTs for initial voiceless stops in elicited words were now a highly significant 75% longer than those for voiced ones, although /tr/ and /dr/ clusters were still not distinguishable. Under the imitation condition, this difference was significantly improved from the elicitation condition to a near normal average of 203%, although the clusters still appeared intractable. Thus there was a significant improvement over the preoperative condition in both the elicitation and the imitation task.

The distinction of final consonant voicing through vowel length showed no improvement over the preoperative condition, however, as Figure 3.10 shows. Vowels in elicited words were in fact more variable in duration than before, rendering the 26% length increase before voiced consonants no longer significant (the single bilabial pair is not distinguished at all). As a result, imitated words were now significantly better than elicited forms, although there was no improvement in what was already an acceptable distinction under imitation conditions before grommet insertion. In fact, although less variable, LS's vowels were now only 41% longer before voiced consonants than before voiceless ones.

## Discussion

In terms of a model of speech processing the cases outlined above can be summarised as follows. In the case of the cleft palate speakers we assume that auditory input is normal and that the input lexicon is therefore also normal. Articulation is initially abnormal because vocal tract structures are abnormal. Once the vocal tract structures have been corrected, there is no immediate change in the output forms. Articulation therapy, using the visual feedback of EPG, provides the means for the speaker to effect such a change. In the case of the glue ear speaker, we must assume that auditory input is not normal. This in turn means that there is no initial voicing distinction represented in the input lexicon, and this can only be developed once hearing has been restored to normal. The main problem which these cases pose for the two-lexicon model lies in the rapidity with which the new forms are adopted.

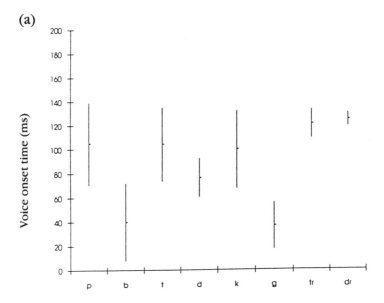

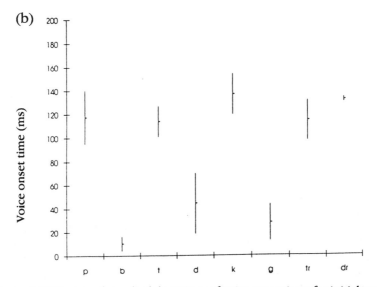

**Figure 3.9** Means and standard deviations of voice onset times for initial stops in the speech of LS after bilateral myringotomy and grommet insertion. (a) in elicitation task (b) in imitation task

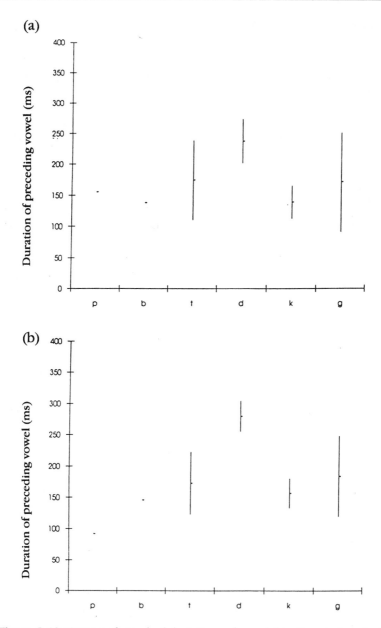

**Figure 3.10** Means and standard deviations of vowel durations before final stops in the speech of LS after bilateral myringotomy and grommet insertion. (a) in elicitation task (b) in imitation task

The cleft palate cases are of particular interest because cleft palate speech is discussed specifically by Hewlett (1990) in relation to his two-lexicon model. As we have seen, he observes that in order to compensate for the anatomical deficit, the motor programmer may either adjust the parameters of the appropriate motor plan – e.g. raise the tongue body – or devise a completely different (from normal) motor plan – e.g.

pharyngeal fricatives as the best achievable correspondence to an /s/ or
/ ʃ / in the input lexicon. In order to be implemented by the 'fast route'
this plan would then be 'phonologised' in the form of an entry in the
output lexicon, with the feature specification [+ PHARYNGEAL], which
would then enable 'semi-automatic' execution of the plan by the motor
processor. Thus Hewlett's model predicts – correctly as it appears – that
'normalisation' of the anatomy by surgical repair would not in itself
result in a change in the articulation of lingual fricatives. However, it also
predicts that such a change can only occur if the speaker consciously
accesses the form(s) afresh from the input lexicon via the 'slow route'
and requires the motor programmer to devise a new plan for its realisation. Only when a new motor plan is 'refined and practised' does it
become part of the mapping rules, thereby bringing about a change in
the representation in the output lexicon. Hewlett stresses that this is a
'gradual revision' of the rules and results in a period of variability in
production. But this prediction of gradual automatisation of a new
motor plan is not easily reconcilable with one aspect of the above cases
which has not been given much emphasis in the reporting: these speakers (and others) mastered the new motor gestures acquired through
visual feedback from the EPG system in a very short period of time (often
in the course of a single session) and typically were able to maintain
these patterns consistently thereafter (F. Gibbon, personal communication). Such outcomes might be more easily accounted for by a model in
which the motor programmer had more direct access to a single lexicon
in which phonological forms were based on (correct) perceptual input,
and in turn served as the basis for motor planning.

The glue ear case is in some ways more complex, in that the impairment appears to lie at the very beginning of the process, at the input
stage. However, there is evidence of some kind of underlying representation of a voicing contrast in final position, although the realisation of
the contrast is inconsistent and inadequate. Nevertheless, there is clearly
no initial contrast in the output lexicon and no motor programme has
been developed to carry it out. In Menn's terms there is a severe output
constraint in LS's speech which limits initial stops in his canonical forms
to a fixed value of the voicing parameter. Once the auditory input is
corrected, we can assume that an initial voicing contrast is developed in
the input lexicon. A motor programme is then devised to produce this
contrast and, once automatised this can be stored in the output lexicon.
However, as with the cleft palate speakers, the acquisition of the contrast
is extremely rapid and largely consistent, and once again this does not
seem to accord with the predictions of the two-lexicon, gradual automatisation model.

A single-lexicon model might more appropriately account for this in
terms of a once-and-for-all connection of a new motor programme with
an existing common underlying representation. This would presuppose

that the final contrast had some kind of representation in the lexicon all along (as it does not rely on acoustic cues which would be likely to be adversely affected by mild high-frequency hearing loss). It would also presuppose that the underlying representation is in the form of a set of contrasting units or features, rather than in the form of canonical structures. We could then hypothesise that the improvement in input enabled the speaker to generalise the contrast to the initial position and to begin fairly rapidly to operate an alternative motor plan (for reduced VOT) to realise the contrast in that position also. The difference in performance in elicitation and imitation tasks indicates that the plan (or its execution) is still not completely mastered. That the less-than-perfect final voicing contrast is itself apparently unaffected by the improvement in input should not surprise us, since high frequency hearing is not involved. But, why was it not adequate to begin with? In normal language acquisition the voicing contrast is acquired later in final position than in initial position. With a common underlying representation in terms of phoneme- or feature-sized units, it is possible that the development of an adequate motor plan for the final contrast was originally in some way inhibited by the lack of input data on the corresponding initial contrast. If so, why did it not proceed once the initial contrast was established? With a single-lexicon single-contrast model, we would have to postulate a variety of contextually determined motor plans for each contrast. Is it possible that the creation of a new plan for a new context is achieved more easily and rapidly than the modification of an existing one? In any case, whether we believe in one lexicon or two, there seems to be a great deal of support for the conclusion that 'old motor plans die hard'.

# References

Dent , H., Gibbon, F. and Hardcastle, W. (1992). Inhibiting an abnormal lingual pattern in a cleft palate child using electropalatography (EPG). In M.M. Leahy and J.K. Kallen (Eds) *Interdisciplinary Perspectives in Speech and Language Pathology*, pp. 211–221. School of Clinical Speech and Language Studies, Trinity College Dublin.

Dodd, B. Leahy, J. and Hambly, G. (1989). Phonological disorders in children: underlying cognitive deficits. *British Journal of Developmental Psychology*, 7, 55–71.

Hardcastle, W., Gibbon, F. and Jones, W. (1991). Visual display of tongue-palate contact: Electropalatography in the assessment and remediation of speech disorders. *British Journal of Disorders of Communication*, 26, 41–74.

Hardcastle, W., Dent, H. and Gibbon, F. (1992). Diagnostic therapy: a case study using electropalatography (EPG). In E. Loebell (Ed.) *Proceedings of the 22nd World Congress of the International Association of Logopedics and Phoniatrics*. Hannover, Germany.

Hardcastle, W., Gibbon, F. and Dent, H. (1994). Assessment and remediation of intractable articulation disorders using EPG. *Annual Bulletin, Research Institute of Logopedics and Phoniatrics*, 27, University of Tokyo, 159–170.

Hewlett, N. (1990). Processes of development and production. In P. Grunwell (Ed.) *Developmental Speech Disorders: Clinical Issues and Practical Implications*, pp. 15–38. Edinburgh: Churchill Livingstone.

Menn, L. (1983). Development of articulatory, phonetic, and phonological capabilities. In B. Butterworth (Ed.) *Language Production*, Vol. 2, pp. 3–50. London: Academic Press.

Smith, N.V. (1973). *The Acquisition of Phonology: A case study*. Cambridge: Cambridge University Press.

Smith, N.V. (1981). On the Cognitive representation of developing phonology. In T.Myers, J.Laver and J.Anderson (Eds) *The Cognitive Representation of Speech*, pp. 313–321. Amsterdam: North Holland.

Waterson, N. (1971). Child phonology: a prosodic view. *Journal of Linguistics*, 7, 179–221.

Waterson, N. (1981). A tentative model of phonological representation. In T. Myers, J. Laver and J. Anderson (Eds) *The Cognitive Representation of Speech*, pp. 323–333. Amsterdam: North Holland.

Williams, N. and Chiat, S. (1993). Processing deficits in children with phonological disorder and delay: a comparison of responses to a series of output tasks. *Clinical Linguistics and Phonetics*, 7, 145–160.

# Chapter 4
# Insights into Language Structure and Function: Some Consequences of Prelingual Hearing Loss

RUTH CAMPBELL

## Abstract

*Studies relating to profound prelingual hearing impairment and the development of language and cognition are reviewed in order to direct speculation concerning the relationship between language and lack of normal (speech) input from birth. The following points are highlighted:*

- *lack of sound input may affect the infant's developing conceptual abilities with as yet unexplored consequences for the development of referential language;*
- *the use of Sign is not a short-cut to language mastery and literacy deserves special attention in this context;*
- *the relationship between gesture, Signed language and spoken language remains opaque.*

*Some ways in which non-linguistic cognitive tasks are performed by people born with profound hearing loss are outlined and some aspects of the biological bases for the development of language and cognition are also sketched in. Overall, study of these children offers no simple insights about either 'Thought without Language', or 'Language without Hearing'. However, when conducted appropriately, studies of cognition and language in people born profoundly hearing impaired can illuminate language processes more generally, as well as pointing to the need for their language to be studied in its own right.*

## Introduction

I will come clean at the outset: when I embarked on some studies of profound prelingual hearing impairment about eight years ago, I did so from the standpoint of a hearing researcher interested in ways in which people with profound prelingual hearing loss may deviate from the normal limits of language use – particularly written language use. My naive assumption was that language deprivation due to early hearing loss would lead to aberrant language skills in a range of domains. In particular, the use of 'inner speech' would be limited in a range of reading, writing and remembering tasks. But the results (e.g. from tasks tapping phonological coding in reading and writing) were not as simple as I thought, while quite different insights emerged as I became more engaged in researching this area. In this chapter I shall sketch some ways in which profound prelingual hearing loss may impact upon language and cognition: some of these are proposals for research, some report work that has been completed. Most of the work reported is not my own. The aim of the chapter is to sketch these areas out sufficiently for the hearing researcher to be aware that the study of language in people with profound prelingual hearing loss may reflect some surprising facets of the language faculty.

To be born without effective hearing has very different implications for language and cognitive function than losing hearing later in life or losing language through cerebral insult. The prognosis for functional language competence is extremely variable and the reasons why one child with impaired hearing will speak well, another one not at all, are still mysterious (Dodd and Murphy, 1992). I shall not attempt to confront this central problem here. One message I shall present is a familiar one: language seems to develop willy-nilly in most people, *as long as the input can deliver the necessary structure*. Where sound is missing, other senses may be put to work to deliver the relevant structural contrasts: these may be visuo-spatial and *sui-generis* (Sign languages); visuo-spatial and parasitic on speech (speechreading; cued speech; forms of Signed spoken language); tactile or polysensory (vibrotactile aids, direct peripheral neural or cortical stimulation). Unless these are available *and* are integrated at the outset into the child's cognitive experience, a child with hearing impairment will be marooned in a world without language.

The second message may be less familiar and is underexplored. The cognitive implications of being born into a world without *sound* – rather than language – remain largely unknown at a time when many developmental psychologists and psycholinguists suggest that the delivery of the world to the child through multisensory channels may be crucial to the formation of shared understanding of how realities and minds are structured. Furthermore, there are conceptual advances in understanding how cognitive structures predate and may prefigure language (Mandler, 1994; Morton, 1994); the role of the sensory input in this initial representational structuring of experience into 'language-sized units' is likely to be critical.

# No sound

Children with profound hearing impairment (hearing loss of > 90 dB in the better ear) are born into a silent world. They do not have access to the many facets of sound; the crack of a glass breaking and the tinkle of its splinters; the thud of a foot on a ball or a fist on a door; the clatter of pans in the kitchen; the cry or song of a beast or person. Not only does this deprive children of direct sensory input (knowing what things 'sound like') but natural exposure to these stimuli confirms the *event-hood* of life; it enables us to parse the world in certain ways. It also enables us to know something of what is 'round the corner' and cannot be seen – it enhances awareness that important things can be displaced from that which is immediately available.

Most direct effects of this simple lack of sensory input have not been systematically explored. One instance: Starkey et al. (1991) have shown that young infants are sensitive to numerosity (doubles, triples, singletons) and that this sensitivity is cross-modal in the earliest months of life. Does this mean that children with hearing impairment, lacking discrete sounds to parse the world into number-based events, are slower than hearing children to pick up on this structure? As far as I know, this has not been investigated. Similarly, no-one has reliably established the consequences for children with hearing impairment that events can never be precipitated 'offscreen', but loom into consciousness only as they enter the field of vision. Mandler (1994) has suggested that, through simple observation and the construction of simple representational schemas, the developing prelingual child is effectively already cutting the world up into chunks that are language-sized. Just how much of this is easy, how much difficult, when sound is missing, is an important and still underexplored question.

Temper tantrums and nervousness in young children with hearing impairment have sometimes been ascribed, by mothers and by clinicians, to the offstage looming of events (see Marschark, 1993, for examples). Nevertheless, it is possible that not only 'cold' cognition (the representation of the inanimate world), but also 'hot' or social cognition (Brothers, 1994) – whereby the child learns about people and how to interact effectively with them – must be easier when all the senses deliver the social world directly to the child. For example, it seems possible that the development of joint attention (Scaife and Bruner, 1975) between child and caregiver depends on spontaneous shared perception of eventhood. If this is askew difficulties in the use of referential pointing and even in the ascription of intentional behaviours may follow. It has been reported that children with hearing impairment are delayed in their ability to perform false belief (theory of mind) tasks (Peterson and Siegal, 1995). While there are a host of reasons why this might be so, it is possible that an initial mismatch between the caregiver and the child's view of what motivates human actions and behaviours could be traced back to difficulties in understanding how events in the world are structured and how people respond to and affect them.

We do know, often from personal reports, that cognitive scotomas relating in surprising ways to lack of sound input can obtain even in adulthood: here is one example.

> My hearing colleague, Helen Wright, worked as a volunteer in a club for people with profound hearing impairment. This also enabled her to maintain a level of competence in Sign (British Sign Language, BSL) which was the members' preferred mode of communication. One young man, Jim, was about to leave for College and did not seem happy about it. 'I'll be lonely there' he confided (in BSL). 'But you'll make friends' said Helen. 'Yes, people will be friendly, I'm sure, but I'll miss the support and warmth of old friends and family', Jim elaborated. 'Have you thought about a pet – a dog, perhaps?', suggested Helen. Jim became distressed. 'No, no, I couldn't have a dog', he insisted. Helen tried to identify why he was so agitated by the idea. None of the usual reasons were the cause of Jim's anguish. Finally he said 'You see, a dog wouldn't understand me'. 'Oh, that's not true,' said Helen, 'After some dog training classes it would be fine'. 'No, no' said Jim 'It's my voice quality: hearing people don't understand me when I speak English, so a dog wouldn't either. And how would I understand what the dog was saying?' Now the penny dropped. Jim believed that dogs spoke and heard English like hearing people. Nothing in his experience suggested that when dogs open their mouths they bark rather than speak. The books he had read and the films he had seen had not put him right: *Watership Down* was full of 'talking' rabbits. This completely unexpected notion had never been disconfirmed by direct experience nor by explicit description.

## No sound – no speech

Seen from the hearing person's perspective, while there may be several consequences of sound loss due to profound hearing impairment, the primary lack is generally, and properly, assumed to be that of normal *speech* input. Children with hearing impairment very rarely develop language abilities at all commensurate with their intelligence. There is increasing evidence that babies become sensitive to some of the segmental characteristics (syllables, stress) of ambient speech before birth and that this tunes them to the sound structure of their native language (Mehler and Christoph, 1994; Kuhl, 1993). Most babies born hearing impaired have sensorineural hearing loss that deprives them of this input as well as heard and spoken speech after birth. Is such loss, itself consequent on sound deprivation from birth or earlier, a necessary and sufficient cause of language failure in people with hearing impairment?

## Born to sign, born to speak: is hearing necessary for language development?

Chomsky famously proposed that language is prefigured. Defined as a rule-governed system whose power (combinatorial, descriptive) resides in the syntax (the combination of words into sentences), it matures in every human individual whose genes permit it to be expressed. This organ of universal grammar (common to all languages) matures in just the same way as do arms, eyes, brains, and requires little in the way of environmental input in order to thrive. Most developmental psycholinguists – closer to the raw data of infant speech – insist, however, that language is both staged and truly formed in accordance with its environment. It is developmental rather than maturational: that is, the constraints imposed by the organism and the environment – perceptual, social, cognitive, emotional – impact directly on the growth of the developing cognitive and linguistic system.

Language development in people with hearing impairment provides support for both an innatist and an empiricist view. Sign languages fit all the requirements for language (e.g. componentiality, duality of patterning, full referentiality) and are grammatically complex: in terms of recent theory (Chomsky, 1981, 1986) current studies suggest that the parameterisation of Sign is identical, formally and developmentally, to that for spoken language. Yet Sign develops on a much smaller ontogenetic and geographical scale than most spoken languages. Very few people are born into a signing world (about 5% of people born hearing impaired, world-wide, have parents with hearing impairment). Those that are generally inhabit small communities. Hearing children of signing parents tend to use speech, not Sign, as a primary language, and there are very few reported cases of second or third generation Sign in hearing offspring of such parents. Thus, Sign generally develops in a 'hostile' environment and has to be renewed in each generation of people with hearing impairment. It is rarely the host language. Sign moreover, has no written form; its culture is entirely in and of itself.

In this context, the viability of Sign and its skilled and fluent practice are especially striking. Children born hearing impaired can acquire Sign as a first language; most of them do not acquire it under anything like 'normal' conditions for language acquisition; their parents are rarely Signers and Sign is largely – though never completely – absent from the world about them. Sign does not develop in a sign-free environment (Feldman, Goldin-Meadow and Gleitman, 1978). There is still uncertainty about the processes whereby Sign develops under such unfavourable circumstances. As with spoken languages, it seems that creolisation occurs in Sign. Where initial models are poor ('sign pidgin'), usually because they are produced by people with speech as a first language, children with hearing impairment elaborate on the initial forms and develop a more componential and flexible system with structured grammatical forms and rich morphology. Indeed in many countries where children with hearing impairment are educated together, Sign develops in school as the children communicate with each other. A number of international programmes are currently exploring the precise ways in which Sign emerges under these conditions.

We know from the work of Bellugi and her colleagues, among others, that adult Sign language can be organised and structured at levels entirely comparable with those of any mature spoken language. A straightforward, but necessarily temporary and contingent conclusion, therefore, is that this provides strong confirmation of Chomsky's claims. Where it develops, Sign is relatively unconstrained by the generally inadequate environment. It requires a medium that allows the comprehension and production of language through a visuo-spatial-gestural channel, and some models of Sign form.

## Without sign: spoken language development without hearing

What, then, of speech? Here a developmental rather than a preformist perspective seems to fit better. While there are some well documented cases of children with hearing impairment who have mastered spoken language 'like a native' (Dodd and Murphy, 1992), most children do not make much progress in the language of the hearing community, remaining resolutely behind their hearing peers at every stage of language comprehension, and showing a widening gap throughout the school years (Rodda and Grove, 1987). Throughout development, their nonverbal IQ, if tested appropriately, remains at chronological age-equivalent levels. Yet children with hearing impairment are surrounded by speakers, and the seen aspects of speech are many and systematic. When speakers talk, their mouths move. Children are sensitive to seen speech movements from birth and this sensitivity is shaped by seen and heard speech within the first four months of life (Dodd, 1979; Kuhl and Meltzoff, 1984).

Why then is it so difficult to pick up speech from the face with little or no residual heard speech? Vision supports effective communication in a variety of ways. When we see people speaking we see referential communication (looking, pointing), turntaking, responsiveness, interruption. We see gestures that are not solely deictic, but subserve other functions (lexical, syntactic, anaphoric): the communicative adequacy of the silent spoken message cannot be gainsaid.

Moreover dynamic aspects of speech, such as rate of speaking and changes in intensity of speech, can be seen as face actions as well as being heard in the acoustic stream. Nevertheless, at strictly segmental (phonological) levels, visual perception of speech can barely support the adequate comprehension of speech content. Fewer than 20% of heard phonemes in English can be reliably distinguished on the lips, so the minimal contrasts that deliver meaning (pin/bin) and morphosyntactic regularities (stay/stayed) are few and far between. Other languages may pose even worse problems for the receiver using speechreading alone: in French, identical liprounding occurs for the acoustically quite different vowels /u/, /o/ and /y/ and sets the lipshape for co-articulated adjacent phonemes, too.

Despite this structural formal difficulty, it is clear that some people born without useful hearing are able to use mouth movements to derive important contrastive information and to follow speech perfectly effectively (Bernstein and Demorest, 1993; Dodd and Murphy, 1992). That is, these good hearing impaired speechreaders must be using some aspects of the seen speech form that can deliver information that is usually understood to be 'invisible' and which is delivered acoustically to people with good hearing. The extent to which such arcana are systematic (that is, are used consistently by different people with hearing impairment) and to what extent they are specific – to particular perceivers and possibly to particular talkers too – remains to be determined. A number of explanations could be proposed: for instance, the kinematics of facial actions can sometimes give information about plosion that is not visible from the still lip-shape itself. Thus the distinction between a seen /m/ and a seen /p/ might be in the visible difference in speed and acceleration of cheek-puffing in the two consonants (Summerfield et al., 1989; Summerfield, 1991). These differences are probably very subtle and, since the distinction between /m/ and /p/ can be picked up relatively easily from the acoustic stream, may not be noticed by hearing speakers of the language. But for the person born hearing impaired, who is sufficiently motivated to be alert to the contrast that is signalled in this way, the difference may be picked up sufficiently well to be useful.

For speechreading to be effective, the speechreader must use context efficiently. A good deal of contextual support is linguistically *intrinsic*. That is, the prediction or interpretation of a particular word or word-segment may depend very heavily on the linguistic interpretation of the message so far. This must be one reason why people with hearing impairment tend to be poorer speechreaders than either hearing people or people with acquired hearing impairment: with less language to start with, they are less able to fill in the gaps where speechreading fails to deliver appropriate contrasts. However, *extrinsic* context is also important in understanding a speaker: where is she looking, and with what expression? People born hearing impaired have no greater problem in using vision to support speech understanding at this level than anyone else. The general point is that without good general language and communication skills, making sense of speech from the lips is a particularly difficult task.

Even when their speech is excellent, people with hearing impairment may still show some anomalies in language use compared with hearing people. Volterra (in press) reports that an Italian woman with excellent speech comprehension and production, nevertheless made reading and writing errors, especially in the omission of articles and some prepositions. She claims that because these particular morphological distinctions are not visible on the lips in Italian they are not as firmly based in this speaker's language as they are in the (spoken and written) language of hearing people. Similarly we have found that in remembering written consonant–vowel lists, students with hearing impairment, who had good oral language, were sensitive to the speechreadability of the lists: lists such as BA, FA, THA, which can be easily discriminated by lipshape, were recalled better than lists such as NA, DA, GA which cannot. No such sensitivity was found for hearing controls (Campbell and Wright, 1989).

Connectionist simulations of language exposure and acquisition (Plunkett, 1993; Plunkett and Marchman, 1993) may provide some help in understanding how an impoverished input can sometimes lead to reasonable language acquisition. Such simulations are urgently required: they should reveal to what extent language delivered in this way may be delayed or deviate from normal patterns, and provide important clues for optimising the input.

## Cued speech: the Brussels experience

When tactile or kinaesthetic support for the missing acoustic distinctions is provided to support speechreading, language comprehension is more likely to develop at near normal levels. A team of researchers at the Free University of Brussels has been investigating a sizeable group of children with profound hearing impairment who have been exposed to cued speech (CS) that supported spoken French (Perier et al., 1987). Around twenty children have been exposed to the system from a very early age (within the first year), a further two dozen on starting school. Cued speech (Cornett, 1967) uses speechreading as the basic system of communication, but words that may be ambiguous in speechreading are disambiguated through synchronised hand gestures. Unlike some other speechreading support systems (e.g. tactile speech), the missing information is not replaced by delivery of the invisible components of lipspeech (primarily invisible *phonetic* features of articulation – for instance vocal cord vibration). Instead, and depending closely on the spoken language, the hands deliver systematic distinctions at a *phonological* level.

The principle that determines the attribution of consonants and vowels to handshapes and hand-positions respectively is that items sharing the same handshape or hand position must be easy to discriminate by speeching. Conversely items difficult to discriminate must belong to different groups. For example a particular hand shape is shared by /p, d, zh/ which are easily discriminated from each other by speeching. Consonants that are difficult to discriminate by speeching like the bilabials /b, p, m/ have different handshapes. The same principle has been used for vowels: a particular hand position is shared by items presenting high discriminability like /i, õ, ã/, and vowels that present similar lipshapes, i.e. the rounded French vowels /y, u, o, õ/ have different hand positions. (Alégria, Charlier and Mattys, 1994)

Note that syllabic structure is indicated systematically; hand position (in space) always indicates a vowel (or diphthong), while handform indicates a consonant. Thus one single gesture indicates a CV, while VC forms require two actions.

Both as an early and a later-acquired system, CS seems to be an effective induction into speech *as long as it is consistently used*. That is, it improves speech understanding in children (Charlier, 1992), with early use giving the greatest advantage. Some very considerable achievements in reading, writing and immediate memory in these children have also been reported, and these literacy-based skills seem to use phonological support in very similar ways to those of hearing children (Alégria et al., 1992; Leybaert, 1993). When it comes to understanding the written word, children with hearing impairment exposed early to CS and the normally hearing child may often be indistinguishable. Furthermore, evidence is accruing that specific syllabic structure of CS leaves a trace in the child's working memory for *written* language: utterances that require several handshape changes (e.g. VCVC forms requiring three or four changes rather than CVCV forms requiring only two) are somewhat more error prone in CS than for speechreading alone.

Do CS users make 'slips of the hand' in repetition? Elicitation studies to date suggest few, if any, hand-only errors. It would seem that these children, like infants acquiring Sign as a first language, attend to both face and hands in an *integrated* way to arrive at the linguistic representation (Snitzer-Reilly et al., 1990). Further studies of CS users will be extremely informative; especially on language production. These children's receptive speech skills are generally very good, but their productive speech can lag. This might be expected since CS affords lexical meanings by mouth shapes and hand signs. While strictly phonological structures are used (lexical differentiation is signalled by seen-and-heard distinctions in mouth shape and hand gesture) this is not how most hearing speakers talk to each other. In order to speak acceptably, children using CS have to find a way to articulate vocally those contrasts to which they are exposed manually and visually. This may be an insuperable difficulty for many children, who prefer to communicate using CS wherever possible. Furthermore, there is sufficient redundancy in the handshapes for CS users to communicate with each other without using lip patterns consistently. Some preliminary evidence from Périer and Alégria's laboratory suggests that early CS users may sometimes ignore the lip-speech pattern in favour of a (conflicting) handshape gesture. A language learned orally may be transmuting into Sign because, paradoxically, this is more suited to the *productive* capacities of the children.

## Newport's hypothesis: when cognition outstrips language development

One well confirmed fact of language acquisition is that there is a critical period in development during which a first language can be acquired effectively. This probably extends up to the end of the seventh year for spoken language. Newport (1990), on the basis of comparative studies of language development in a variety of different groups including people with hearing impairment, suggests that the mechanism for language acquisition in childhood is determined by the child's initial sampling strategy, which is itself constrained by memorial and perceptual limitations. Because of these limitations, infants and young children can only grasp some aspects of the language to which they are exposed. This part-sampling strategy allows the development of sensitivity to regularities in language (to phonotactic and morphosyntactic rules). A similar claim was put forward by Pettito and Seidenberg (1979) in the context of monkeys and language. They argued that monkeys were too smart, too young, to develop language. A similar principle underlies some neural-net modelling of the acquisition of some regular inflectional forms, where a small hidden-unit layer between input and output forces regularisation learning.

In the language-deprived, including many people born hearing impaired, and in late (but not young) second language learners, rather different mechanisms are used. More mature perceptual and memorial systems lead to a different processing mode: language acquired in this way may be relatively rich in vocabulary, yet lack fully realised syntactic and phonological structures. There are similarities between the patterns of language acquisition of children with hearing impairment and (late) second language learners. For example, both groups appear to be particularly deficient in morphosyntactic skills. However, the language deficits of children with hearing impairment are not confined to syntactic and morphological aspects: vocabulary lags, too, and semantic skills may not be good (Dodd, McIntosh and Woodhouse, in press). Many current approaches stress the *interaction* between vocabulary, syntactic and semantic acquisition processes (Gleitman and Gillette; 1995, Bowerman, 1994). While insights into the mechanisms governing the structure of the critical period for the normal acquisition of language may be gleaned from people with hearing impairment, these insights still need to be convincingly integrated.

## Second language learning, speechreading and literacy

Newport reminds us that language is not necessarily learned once and early. Its acquisition may be extended over many years or different languages may be learned after the mother tongue. The older child or adult has another way into language, one based on explicit training and problem solving. Literacy is not acquired as a native language but in this 'second language' way. It is noteworthy that, in all cultures, literacy training begins at the age at which mastery of spoken language is assumed to be secure. For people born hearing impaired and with poor command of either speech or Sign, I have suggested that literacy can form an important route into language mastery (Campbell, in press). Unlike hearing children, the problem for children with hearing impairment, on being faced with their first reading book, is not to map the squiggles to words 'in his head', but to use the squiggles to fill in holes in their language knowledge. Those with Sign as a first language have a horrendous problem on encountering written speech, and, unsurprisingly, rarely achieve literacy levels commensurate with their (signed) language skills (Marschark and Harris, 1995). Their task is equivalent to a child with English as a first language learning to read and write in Chinese, not knowing what spoken Chinese may be like and never having learned to read and write in English. Writing systems have evolved (albeit in their different ways) to rest upon the shoulders of the spoken language that begot them; they are not designed to mediate between languages.

Some of the implications of this difficulty are starting to be understood. In Britain, it had long been assumed that the poor written language of children with hearing impairment reflected their poor basic language skills. Now, however, we can see that, quite often, written English by these writers simply betrays its Sign origins. Here are two examples from a recent study of the spontaneous writing errors of 'bilingual' children with hearing impairment (Gregory, in press). The writers' linguistic upbringing comprised some Sign, though not necessarily in the home or from an early age, and some exposure to speech.

1. *Fire Pink Panther throw water to the fire*

   This follows the topic–comment structure of BSL ([fire]–[Pink Panther]–[throw]), rather than the SVO structure of English. But in addition the child adds in some SVO ordering, too ('water to the fire). A 'belt and braces' approach that suggests high levels of metalinguistic skill, but some unsureness about the correct forms.

2. *I drive arrive*

   In BSL, Finish (the aspect of language that shows that a topic has ended) is signed by a form that can be lexically translated as 'arrive'. In written English, of course, a punctuation point is used. This child has not yet learned the appropriate *form* to use in writing.

These 'errors' of written language suggest that the road from Sign to reading is quite rocky. There is, however, no reason to be too pessimistic about the ability of children with hearing impairment to access reading from speech. Their ability to phonologically decode (ascribe letters to word-sounds) can be good (Dodd, 1979). Time and again, in studies with teenagers who are hearing impaired, I have found that although their reading comprehension is poor, they are not particularly impaired in mapping letters to sounds. They tend to perform more-or-less on a par with reading-age matched readers and writers on reading and spelling tasks (Burden and Campbell, 1995). These children are exposed to speech in the real world and are often drilled at school in both phonics for reading and writing and in using a hearing aid to distinguish speech sounds. However, while their level of phonological *awareness* is high, their level of phonological *skill* may be lower.

Bilingualism in speech and Sign may offer the best chance for children with hearing impairment to master reading and writing. Sign may deliver the rich conceptual world for which children who lack Sign have to struggle, and speech has an important complementary role because it is closer to the written word than is Sign. Although segmental contrasts cannot be perceived reliably from mouth actions, nevertheless speech has the potential to deliver the decoding rules for making sense of the printed page.

## Gesture, Sign and speech in development

The relationship between gestural communication and the development of Sign in people with hearing impairment, and speech in hearing people is an important one, which is still underexplored in cognitive terms (McNeill, 1985). Claims that language developed from manual gesture systems have existed since such matters started to be discussed scientifically. Some researchers claim that Sign is a linguistic medium from its first appearance. Bonvillian and Folven (1993) suggest that for children exposed to Sign as a first language, early discrete hand movements, which have lexical status, can occur at around the sixth month, predating the hearing child's first words. Continuing the theme of 'the primacy of Sign', Pettito and Marentette (1994), in a study of hearing and hearing impaired children of signing parents, have claimed that mabbling (manual babbling) both predates and extends the timespan of hearing children's spoken syllabic babbling. According to these researchers, such manual-play can extend well into the second year. For researchers like Pettito, if Sign is available to the infant in early life, it develops as a language *ab initio*; mabbling shows the child engaging directly with the segmental structure of this language.

In contrast to this viewpoint is a more integrated perspective. Over the past fifteen years Volterra (in press) has examined the relationship between gesture and language development in young children with hearing impairment acquiring Sign and control children. How do their communication skills and their language skills overlap, how diverge? Two types of gestural communication can be seen by around 10 months of age in both groups of children: deixis (pointing, giving) and representational gestures (mimetic forms e.g. greetings such as 'bye-bye', objects like 'phone'). At this age, children's communication abilities may appear to be in advance of their language skills. However, while for hearing children these forms 'freeze' as spoken language develops further, this is not so for children with hearing impairment, whose communication needs are not met by their generally slow language development. They continue to use gesture over the next year, and it becomes extended and integrated with developing speech *or* Sign. During this period, however, only some combinations of gesture and word are observed. In particular, gestural representations (e.g. for objects) are *never* combined with language-based ones, while deictic gestures may be. In children learning Sign as a first language, early gestures appear to be incorporated into the acquisition of Sign forms, but in a linguistically constrained manner (see also, Pettito, 1987).

Volterra suggests that this implies a *common* basis for the development of language, gesture and Sign: language (and other cognitive skills) become modularised during development, rather than being delivered in ready-made modular packets. This view appears to be supported by studies of children with brain lesions in early life: some cognitive competence always precedes language use – in both right and left hemispherectomised infants. Whether this view will appear so persuasive when other special groups are investigated (e.g. youngsters with autism, Williams syndrome) awaits research.

Studies of gesture – in relation both to speech and Sign – are part of the larger enterprise of gaining understanding of the cognitive models ('representations', Morton, 1994) onto which language maps. I will now turn to this aspect of cognition in people with hearing impairment: are there special ways in which they think that reflects their idiosyncratic language development?

# Some things the people with hearing impairment (may) do better

### Perspective taking

Children receiving Sign have to shift perspective to that of the Signer in order to produce the signed message. That is, they must reverse events in the person-to-person plane where signing takes place. In learning Sign, while signing mothers sometimes form children's signs directly, by manipulating their hands while standing behind or beside them, the commonest form of learning is confrontational. This leaves a mark on developing spatial abilities. Where Sign is a first language it is quite likely that there is a perspective-taking advantage over hearing children in interpreting movements in space. For example, Pettito (1987) has elegantly shown how deictic reference is interpreted by children with hearing impairment in relation to the speaker, not the receiver (and that this use develops in a very similar manner to the hearing child's use of the similar shifting reference pronouns, 'me' and 'you'). Lateral (left–right) inversion of gestures, too, is correctly performed by early Signers, but can be particularly problematic for learners of Sign as a second language.

But does perspective-taking skill extend beyond the language domain? One recent study (Masataka 1995) suggests that children with Sign as a first language are better than age-matched hearing controls at reporting the 'correct' (i.e. producer-viewpoint) orientation of tactile forms like letters 'drawn' on the perceiver's forehead, which most recipients perceive as mirror-reversed (Corcoran, 1977). Three-year-olds, both hearing impaired and hearing, performed like hearing adults, and were susceptible to a mirror illusion. However, four-year-old children with hearing impairment who were mastering Sign, showed flexibility and power in interpreting the drawn form. For example, they might ask, 'Which way do you want me to say it? How it looks to you, or to me?' The illusion had no power over them.

This field is open for further systematic exploration in the domain where cognition and language overlap. For example, some action terms are particularly hard to learn; these include those where thematic roles are reversed (give/take; borrow/lend; rent/lease). Typically these are acquired late by hearing children (Clark, 1995) and are often susceptible to damage in aphasia. But since children acquiring Sign learn perspective taking in propositional settings from an early age, and such forms require clear positional analysis, they may be better at this task than non-Signing children of similar language competence.

### Immediate memory – more space, less sound

O'Connor and Hermelin (1978) showed that subjects with hearing impairment, given the choice of remembering list items in spatial or temporal order, chose spatial ordering. This finding, however, does not readily replicate: moreover it is far from simple to set up a task where spatial and temporal ordering choices are fully separable (see Hanson, 1982). Less contentiously, a child with hearing impairment is less a 'slave to the spoken word' in recall than a comparable hearing child. In our work, for example, we found that children with hearing impairment tended to be better than hearing children at random paired-associate picture learning, but worse at learning rhyme-based picture pairs. They tended not to use names to prop up picture recall and, when they did, were somewhat less affected by word homophony. However, there was no sign that these subjects sidestepped phonological coding when *written* material was to be processed. If anything, their reading, writing and remembering resembled that of much younger hearing children in its dependence on speech-structured forms (Campbell, 1992).

### Enhanced visuo-spatial skills?

Bellugi and colleagues have explored non-linguistic cognitive abilities in skilled Signers. They theorised that spatial cognitive skills may be extended in these people because of the spatial requirements of Sign and found that, on a number of cognitive tasks, Signers outperformed matched hearing controls (Bellugi et al., 1990). These were tasks of visuo-spatial competence, including face processing across different views and Block design. One particularly impressive feat was the spatial analysis of dynamic displays. Subjects were required to replicate forms ('Chinese letters') drawn by a point light-source on a screen. That is, the 'nonsense form' had to be constructed from the fading display. People with hearing impairment outperformed their hearing peers conclusively. The task, as Bellugi indicates, draws on precisely those spatio-dynamic skills required to analyse Sign input, yet it was not in the language domain. Of further note, the advantage was most evident in the younger (3–5) age groups, just as in the perspective-taking experiment cited above. Is this an example of *perceptual* 'sharpening' in people who sign? If so, might this mean that their brains become organised in a radically different way than those of children who speak? The last ten years have seen some important progress in understanding the neurological and neuropsychological bases of Sign and of cognition in people with hearing impairment more generally. These are now briefly considered.

# Sign neuropsychology and space in sign

The neuropsychology of Sign is now well established. Following the pioneering study of six case studies of native ASL Signers who had suffered localised lesions (Poizner et al., 1986) it was clear that Sign is localised in a manner analogous to spoken language, and more recent investigations confirm this pattern. Aphasia and apraxia dissociate in Sign as in spoken language. Left hemisphere lesions affect both the perception and reception of Sign, but fail to affect either non-linguistic gesture or other cognitive abilities. By contrast, right-sided lesions spare language function but affect visuo-spatial competence. There was just one indication of 'overlap' between processing requirements and localisation: a patient with right-sided (parietal?) damage showed deficits in the use of the syntactic Sign space: this showed a skewing and a shrinking to the right, analogous to neglect in reading and writing in hearing patients.

## Is spatialised syntax arbitrary?

Spatialised syntax is one of the unique features of Sign: reference to events is made by movements and by referential gesture (including pointing and looking) in a defined area in front of the producer, and these are construed syntactically by the receiver. However, the Sign-linguist, Scott Lidell, has pointed out that, far from being arbitrary in its mappings from space to language, Sign constrains itself to specific spatial relationships in a topographic space that is not intrinsically linguistic. Liddell argues that the mapping space used to display Sign utterances and gestural or visual maps used by spoken language users to communicate, for example, the position of the hairdresser's shop in relation to the butcher's, are *identical* in format and constraints. Moreover, however linguistic may be the use of particular tokens to designate events, agents or locales, they nevertheless obey 'natural' topographic rules that are extra-linguistic. Reference to the top of a building or object in Sign must be to the top of the token; where classifiers (unique Sign constructions that maintain reference throughout an utterance) are used, their topography is the 'natural' one, and not one that is imposed by an arbitrary linguistic form. For example, if people are referred to by an upright index finger they have a 'front' and a 'back' that cannot be violated ('she followed him' must involve appropriate positioning of the indicators).

Sign has no way of referring to spatialised events without such structures. The precise development and breakdown of these spatially-sensitive forms is not yet evident. For instance, might right parietal damage (which can affect spatial location abilities) impair *some* aspects of spatialised language? Neuropsychological studies to date only suggest that the syntactic Sign space may be distorted (just as such patients may show neglect in reading or writing), not that the forms themselves are misused.

## Developmental issues

Sign localises much like speech in the adult brain (although our knowledge is still extremely fuzzy concerning some crucial aspects of spatial and linguistic representation). But how do such specialisations develop? To what extent are brain structures preformed to subserve specific functions; to what extent does experience modulate the final location and character of these functions? There are a number of possibilities concerning such neural and functional plasticity – particularly in respect of visual function – in relation to hearing impairment: some of these are sketched below.

### What develops fastest, first? Structures?

De Schonen (de Schonen et al., 1993) has claimed that the initial development of the right hemisphere is in advance of that of the left hemisphere. Others have claimed, in complementary fashion, that the left hemisphere is particularly sensitive to developmental insult (e.g. from variations in peripuerperal hormone levels, Geschwind and Galaburda, 1986). A further suggestion is that this differential speed of development 'sets' the right hemisphere to function best to its earliest specifications. These are for low spatial frequency and for fast, global analysis in contrast to the more fine-grain, slower analysis by left hemisphere mechanisms.

### What develops fastest, first? Functions?

Neurophysiological research has shown that dorsal and ventral visual processing streams have been identified which specialise in different functional analyses of (primarily visual) input (the 'what' and 'where' systems; Ungerleider and Mishkin, 1982). It has been suggested that the 'where' system (the parietal stream) completes development by the age of two years, while the 'what' (infero-temporal) system continues to develop through childhood (Vital-Durand, Atkinson and Braddick, 1995). If we map this functional insight onto the lateralisation proposals, this suggests that the development of a number of right hemisphere based functions – especially those that are space-based (orientation, manipulation of objects, possibly face recognition) – may be relatively complete by early childhood, in relation to left hemisphere based functions, which may mature more slowly and also show greater vulnerability to derailment through development. Most developmental laterality studies support this generalisation.

### What develops best: Action-based systems?

In contrast to the extensive speculation concerning perceptual plasticity, the possibility has not yet been addressed that more anterior structures, related to the production of Sign (or of speech) may be differently localised and show different time-courses of development in people with hearing impairment than in hearing people. Manual productions are localised in left anterior structures, just as are speech-articulatory ones. But the space-constraints on Sign are quite different than those for speech and the involvement of parietal systems, particularly those that may be linked to perception-for-action (Goodale and Milner, 1992) have not yet been explored.

### Sensory loss and functional compensation

At all events, the effects of loss of hearing on the relative rate of development of different processing streams and of different functional specialisations is an important topic for further research. Physiological evidence points to 'dieback' of a large number of primary sensory neurones as part of the tuning of the newborn animal to environmental contingencies. How much further might this extend (into putative secondary association cortex areas) in people with hearing impairment? Studies with small mammals show some reorganisation of auditory cortex following *unilateral* section of the auditory nerve, and it is likely that auditory receptive cortex may be colonised by afferents from other areas if it is not innervated in the normal manner.

Neville and Lawson (1987) studied evoked brain potentials for the detection of simple visual targets in people with Sign as a first language. One of their major findings is that these hearing impaired subjects show more marked visual evoked potentials to peripheral visual events (visual flashes) than do hearing people, and they speculate that this is *directly* due to auditory sensory loss – a form of neural compensation. They also found laterality differences between the two groups. Whereas hearing subjects showed greater amplitude differences and more activity in the right hemisphere for this task, the advantage switched to the left hemisphere in the hearing impaired group. This appears to be due to the acquisition of left hemispheric specialisation for Sign (Poizner, Battison and Lane, 1979), for they report a similar asymmetry in hearing children of Signing parents.

Neville's work therefore alerts us to two aspects of cortical specialisation in congenital absence of hearing: direct sensory reorganisation of cortical receptive areas and function-specific reorganisation, dependent on the acquisition of Sign. But experiments similar to these have not been carried out with people with hearing impairment for whom Sign is not a primary language, and this (together with other non-invasive studies of cortical localisation) is an imperative for further research, if we are to understand how function and structure relate in terms of neural plasticity.

## Coming round

Research in profound prelingual hearing loss is changing. While this review has taken a hearing researcher's viewpoint – and something of a neuroscientific one at that – the culture of people with hearing impairment is imposing its own agenda on that of linguists, psychologists and other professionals. In forthcoming years their education and welfare will take a number of new turns, as the people with hearing impairment identify their own needs and rights within hearing and speaking societies. In turn, this will impact on the education and development of new generations of people born with hearing impairment. Add to this the potential impact of widespread cochlear implant programmes, to 'cure deafness', and only the most clairvoyant would hazard any predictions concerning the research questions that will be important in five, ten or fifteen years time. Against this changing background, I have attempted a whistle-stop tour of some recent landmarks in research in hearing impairment. Its aim has been to identify areas likely to be fruitful in advancing our understanding of the mechanisms of language, of its relations to cognition, and of the brain substrates that support these.

How then does profound hearing impairment illuminate normal language function? The following points are the important ones to hold:

*Variability in language exposure and upbringing is the key characteristic of profound prelingual hearing impairment.*

We do not yet know to what extent the lack of sound rather than the lack of speech may colour the development of cognition. People born hearing impaired rarely have access to early Sign, and visible speech (speechreading), which does surround them, does not usually deliver sufficient contrastive information for language to develop normally. However it is a relatively simple matter to *augment* speechreading, and when this is done systematically, receptive language can improve dramatically. While cued speech is one such example, the acquisition of literacy in the spoken language may also be considered to be a way of delivering the 'invisible' aspects of speech. Although this is necessarily taught rather than acquired as a first language, it can, nevertheless, help to deliver the important contrasts that delineate the spoken language. People with Sign may show evidence of its structure in their reading and writing performance and in spoken language – just as other bilinguals do (and as several chapters in this volume suggest) – and this may be a problem, but not an insuperable one, in making literacy work for people with hearing impairment, who show high levels of phonological awareness without necessarily showing good phonological skills.

*Sign appears to be able to deliver a first language more readily and more completely than does speech.*

However, this supposition may yet be overturned: to date, most of the widely cited studies have been on people with Sign acquired early from good models. What we know about Sign is that it is linguistically structured and represented in the brains of Signers as speech is in hearing brains. However, there are still a large number of unknown aspects of Sign: how does it originate; can everyone acquire it; how does it relate to the use of gesture? The unique features of Sign may prove less tractable to the simple notion that it is a language 'like any other'. In particular, the special use of space in Sign (in syntax, in the use of classifiers and reference) will bear a great deal of further psychological and neurological interrogation.

## Conclusion

Does the study of hearing impairment offer direct insights into the structure of language and its development? Only up to a point: the studies of the last fifteen years have shown that language in a visuo-gestural medium can develop systematically when hearing is absent, and that some reorganisation of other cognitive and cortical functions may follow from this. But further inferences are not simple, and many findings have uncovered more questions than they have answered. The relationships between gesture and language, and the autonomy of language itself (how does it interface with spatial and conceptual cognition?) loom more problematically than ever. The circumstances under which one child with hearing impairment will understand and use speech while another one cannot (and will not) is still mysterious. However these questions are addressed, the answers are unlikely to be quite those we expect.

## Acknowledgements

Preparation of this work was supported by the Leverhulme Trust; the Economic and Social Research Council of Great Britain, through a seminar series on **Cognition and Deafness**; and by the University of Queensland (travel award). I also thank the Cognition and Deafness Research group, especially Bencie Woll, Sue Gregory, Marc Marschark, Jesus Alégria, Jacqueline Leybaert, Margaret Harris, John Clibbens and Mairead MacSweeney for discussions.

## References

Alégria, J., Leybaert, J., Charlier, B. and Hage, C. (1992). On the origin of phonological representations in the deaf: hearing lips and hands. In J. Alégria, D. Holender, J. Morais and M. Radeau (Eds) *Analytic Approaches to Human Cognition*. Amsterdam: Elsevier, North Holland.

Alégria, J., Charlier, B. and Mattys, S. (1994). The role of lipreading and cued speech on the processing of phonological information in deaf children. Unpublished ms., *Lab de Psychologie Experimentale*, ULB, Brussels, Belgium.

Bates, E., Dale, P.S. and Thal, D (1995). Individual differences and their implications for theories of language development. In P. Fletcher and B. MacWhinney (Eds) *The Handbook of Child Language*, pp. 96–151. Oxford: Blackwell.

Bellugi, U., O'Grady, L., Lillo-Martin, D., O'Grady Hynes, M, van Hoek, K and Corina, D. (1990). Enhancement of spatial cognition in deaf children. In V. Volterra and C. Erting (Eds) *Gesture to Language in Hearing and Deaf Children*, pp. 279–303. London: Springer.

Bernstein, L.E. and Demorest, M.E. (1993). Speech perception without audition. *Journal of the Acoustical Society of America*, **94**, 1887.

Bonvillian, J. and Folven, R. J. (1993). Sign language acquisition: developmental aspects. In M. Marscharck and M.D. Clark (Eds) *Psychological Perspectives on Deafness*, pp. 229–265. Hillsdale, N.J.: Erlbaum.

Bowerman, M. (1994). Early grammatical development. *Philosophical Transactions of the Royal Society of London*, B, **346**, 37–46.

Brothers, L. (1994). Neurophysiology of the perception of intentions by primates. In M. Gazzaniga (Ed.) *The Cognitive Neurosciences*, pp. 1107–1115. Cambridge: MIT.

Burden, V. and Campbell, R. (1995) Phonological awareness, reading and spelling in the profoundly deaf. In B. de Gelder and J. Morais (Ed.) *Phonological Awareness and Literacy: Comparative Approaches*, pp. 109–124. Hove, UK: Erlbaum.

Campbell, R. (in press). Read the lips: Speculations on cognitive and academic development in prelingual deafness. In M. Marschaick, P. Siple, D. Lillo Martin, V. Eberhart and R. Campbell. *Relations of Language and Cognition: The View from Sign Language and Being Deaf.* Oxford: Oxford University Press.

Campbell, R. (1992). Speech in the head? Rhyme skill, reading and immediate memory in the deaf. In D. Reisberg (Ed.) *Auditory Imagery*, pp. 73–94. Hillsdale, N.J.: Erlbaum..

Campbell, R. and Wright, H. (1989). Immediate memory in the orally-trained deaf: effects of 'lipreadability' in the recall of written syllables. *British Journal of Psychology*, **80**, 299–312.

Campbell, R. and Wright, H. (1990). Deafness and immediate memory for pictures: dissociations between inner speech and the inner ear? *Journal of Experimental Child Psychology*, **50**, 259–286.

Charlier, B. (1992). Complete Signed and cued French. *American Annals of the Deaf*, **137**, 331–337.

Chomsky, N. (1970). Reading, writing and phonology. *Harvard Educational Review*, **40**, 287–311.

Chomsky, N. (1981). *Lectures on Government and Binding*, Dordrecht, Boston: Kluwer.

Chomsky, N. (1986). *Knowledge of Language; its nature origins and use*, London: Praeger.

Clark, E.V. (1995). Later lexical development and word formation. In P. Fletcher and B. MacWhinney (Eds) *The Handbook of Child Language*, pp. 393–411. Oxford: Blackwell.

Corcoran, D.W. J. (1977). The phenomenon of the disembodied eye (or is it a matter of personal geography?). *Perception*, **6**, 247–253.

Cornett, O. (1967). Cued Speech. *American Annals of the Deaf*, **112**, 3–13.

De Schonen, S., Deruelle, C., Mancini, J. and Pascalis, O. (1993). Hemispheric differences in face processing and brain maturation. In B. de Boysssons-Bardies., S. de Schonen, P. Juzscyck, P. McNeilage. and J. Morton. (Eds) *Developmental Neurocognition: Speech and face processing in the first year of life*, pp. 149–164. Dordrecht, Boston: Kluwer.

Dodd, B. (1979). Lipreading in infants: attention to speech presented in and out of synchrony. *Cognitive Psychology*, **11**, 478–484.

Dodd, B. and Murphy, J. (1992). Visual Thoughts. In R. Campbell (Ed.) *Mental Lives: Case studies in Cognition*. Oxford: Blackwell.

Dodd, B., McIntosh, B. and Woodhouse, L. (in press). The acquisition of speechreading by profoundly prelingually hearing-impaired children. In D. Stork (Ed.) *Speech Reading in Machine and Humans: A NATO ISI Meeting*. Springer.

Feldman, H., Goldin-Meadow, S. and Gleitman, L. (1978). Beyond Herodotus: the creation of language by linguistically deprived deaf children. In A. Lock (Ed.) *Action, Symbol and Gesture: The Emergence of Language*. New York: Academic Press.

Geschwind, N. and Galaburda, A. M. (1986). Cerebral lateralization: biological mechanisms (II). *Archives of Neurology*, **42**, 521–552.

Gleitman, L. and Gillette, J. (1995). The role of syntax in verb learning. In P. Fletcher and B. MacWhinney (Eds) *The Handbook of Child Language*, pp. 413–428. Oxford: Blackwell.

Goodale, M. and Milner, A D. (1992). Separate visual pathways for perception and action. *TINS*, **15**, 20–24.

Gopnik, M. and Crago, M. (1991). Familial aggregation of a developmental language disorder. *Cognition* **39**, 1–50.

Green, K. and Miller, J. (1985). On the role of visual rate information in phonetic perception. *Perception and Psychophysics*, **38**, 269–276.

Gregory, S. (in press). Bilingualism in sign and speech: effects on written productions. *Proceedings of the 1995 Child Language Symposium*, Bristol, April.

Hanson, V.L. (1982). Short-term recall by deaf Signers of American Sign Language: Implications of encoding strategy for order recall. *Journal of Experimental Psychology: Learning, Memory and Cognition*, **8**, 572–583.

Jusczyk, P.W., Hirsh-Pasek, K., Kemler Nelson, D.G., Kennedy, L.J., Woodward, A. and Piwoz, J. (1992). Perception of acoustic correlates of major phrasal units by young infants. *Cognitive Psychology*, **24**, 252–293.

Kuhl, P. (1993). Developmental speech perception: implications for models of language development. *Annals of the NY Academy of Sciences*, **682**, 248–263.

Kuhl, P. and Meltzoff, A. (1984). The intermodal representation of speech in infancy. *Science*, **218**, 1138–1141.

Leybaert, J. (1993). Reading ability in the deaf. In M. Marschark and D. Clark (Eds) *Psychological Perspectives in Deafness*,. New York: Erlbaum.

Lidell, S. (1994). *Conceptual and Linguistic Issues in Spatial Mapping: comparing spoken and signed language* (Unpublished paper, Gallaudet University).

Mandler, J. (1994). Precursors of linguistic knowledge. *Philosophical Transactions of the Royal Society of London*, **B**, 346, 63–69.

Marschark, M. (1993). *Psychological Development of Deaf Children*. New York: Oxford University Press.

Marschark, M. and Harris, M. (1995). Success and failure in learning to read: the special case(?) of deaf children. In J. Oakhill and C. Cornoldi (Eds) *Reading Comprehension Disabilities: Processes and Intervention*. Hillsdale, N.J.: Lawrence Erlbaum.

Masataka, N. (1995). Decentralisation and absence of mirror reversal tendency in cutaneous pattern perception of deaf children. *British Journal of Developmental Psychology*

McNeill, D. (1985). So you think gestures are non-verbal? *Psychological Review*, **92**, 350–371.

Mehler, J. and Christoph, A. (1994). Language in the infant's mind. *Philosophical Transactions of the Royal Society of London*, **B**, 346, 13–20.

Morton, J. (1994). Language and its biological context. *Philosophical Transactions of the Royal Society of London*, **B**, 346, 5–13.

Neville, H. and Lawson, D. (1987). Attention to central and peripheral visual space in a movement detection task: an event-related potential and behavioral study I: Hearing subjects; II Congenitally deaf adults. *Brain Research*, **405**, 253–267; 268–283.

Neville, H.J., Kutas, M. and Schmidt, A. (1982). ERP studies of cerebral specialisation during reading congenitally deaf adults. *Brain and Language*, **16**, 316–337.

Newport, E. (1990). Maturational constraints on language learning. *Cognitive Science*, **14**, 11–28.

O'Connor, N. and Hermelin, B. (1978). *Seeing and Hearing in Space and Time*. London: Academic Press.

Périer, O., Charlier, B., Hage, C. and Alégria, J. (1987). Evaluation of the effects of prolonged cued-speech practice on the perception of spoken language. In I.G.Taylor (Ed.) *The Education of the Deaf: current perspectives*,Vol 1. International Congress on Education for the Deaf, Beckenham, Kent, UK (Croom-Helm).

Peterson, C. and Siegal, M. (1995). Deafness, conversation and theory of mind. *Journal of Psychology, Psychiatry and Allied Disciplines*, **36**, 459 474.

Pettito, L.A. (1987). On the autonomy of language and gesture: evidence from the acquisition of personal pronouns in American Sign Language. *Cognition*, **27**, 1–52.

Pettito, L.A. and Marentette, P.F. (1994). Babbling in the manual mode: evidence for the ontogeny of language. *Science*, **251**, 1493–1496.

Pettito, L.A. and Seidenberg, M. (1979). On the evidence for linguistic abilities in Signing apes. *Brain and Language*, **8**, 162–183.

Plunkett, K. (1993). Lexical segmentation and vocabulary growth in early language acquisition. *Journal of Child Language*, **20**, 43–60.

Plunkett, K. and Marchman, V. (1993). From rote learning to system building: acquiring verb morphology in children and connexionist nets. *Cognition*, **48**, 21–69.

Poizner, H., Battison, R. and Lane, H. (1979). Cerebral asymmetries for American Sign Language: the effects of moving stimuli. *Brain and Language*, **7**, 351–362.

Poizner, H., Klima, E. and Bellugi , U. (1986). *What the Hands Reveal to the Brain*. Cambridge: MIT Press.

Rodda, M. and Grove, C. (1987). *Language, Cognition and Deafness*. Hillsdale, N.J.: Erlbaum.

Scaife, M. and Bruner, J. (1975). The capacity for joint visual attention in the infant. *Nature*, **253**, 265–266.

Snitzer-Reilly, J., McIntire, M.L. and Bellugi, U. (1990). Faces: the relationship between language and affect. In V. Volterra and C.J. Erting (Eds) *From Gesture to Language in Hearing and Deaf Children*. Berlin: Springer.

Starkey, P., Spelke, E. and Gelman, R. (1991). Numerical abstraction by human infants. *Cognition*, **36**, 97–127.

Summerfield, A.Q. (1991). The visual perception of phonetic gestures. In I.G. Mattingley and M. Studdert-Kennedy (Eds) *Modularity and the Motor Theory of Speech Perception: Proceedings of a Conference to Honour Alvin M. Liberman*. Hillsdale, N.J.: Lawrence Erlbaum.

Summerfield, A.Q., McLeod, A., McGrath, M. and Brooke, M. (1989). Lips, teeth and the benefits of lipreading. In A.W. Young and H.D. Ellis (Eds) *Handbook of Research in Face Processing*. pp. 218–223. Amsterdam: North Holland.

Ungerleider, L.G. and Mishkin, M. (1982). Two cortical visual systems. In D.J. Ingle, M.A. Goodale and R.J.W. Mansfield (Eds) *Analysis of Visual Behaviour*, pp. 549–586. Cambridge: MIT Press.

Vital-Durand, F., Atkinson, J. and Braddick, O. (1995). *Infant Vision*, pp. 327–344. Oxford: OUP.

Volterra, V. (in press). Gesture, hearing impairment and language development. *Proceedings of the 1995 Child Language Symposium*.

# Chapter 5
# Individual Differences in Cognitive Function among Normal Subjects and their Implications for Cognitive Neuropsychology

RANDI C. MARTIN

## Abstract

*This chapter discusses the implications for cognitive neuropsychological research of individual differences in the performance of normal subjects. Before direct consideration of this issue, the assumptions of the cognitive neuropsychological approach are briefly laid out with regard to the manner in which patient data are analysed. With this background in mind, the discussion focuses on whether variation in normal subjects' performance challenges the assumptions underlying the analysis of patient data.*

## Introduction

In cognitive neuropsychology, an information processing approach is taken to the analysis of a cognitive domain such as memory, language or object recognition in that performance is assumed to be dependent on the operation of a system of cognitive components (see Ellis and Young, 1987; Shallice, 1988, for overviews of work taking this approach). These components are assumed to consist of different types of mental representations (e.g. orthographic, semantic) and processes for mapping between these representations (e.g. mapping between a visual–spatial representation and a semantic representation in object naming). The components are organised into a processing system such that information flows between these components in certain directions but not others (e.g. a visual–spatial representation connects to a semantic representation but not directly to a phonological representation). Brain damage may affect any of these components separately, with the result that performance depends on the operation of the remaining components.

In studying brain-damaged patients, the goal is to determine which cognitive components have been affected and which preserved. Often the pattern of results provides new information on the nature of the cognitive components involved in a given domain by demonstrating unexpected dissociations – that is, good performance on some tasks despite very impaired performance on others. For example, Warrington and Shallice (1969) reported on the patient KF who, despite having a very restricted short-term memory capacity (i.e. a memory span of about one item), showed normal long-term learning on a variety of standard tasks. Such findings went against theories current at the time which assumed that the amount of time that information was held in short-term memory predicted long-term learning. More generally, cognitive neuropsychological findings have provided important insights into the nature of the organisation of cognitive domains.

The cognitive neuropsychological approach entails case study methodology, in which patients are examined individually (see Caramazza, 1984; Caramazza and McCloskey, 1988 for discussion). Aside from a thorough examination of each patient, there are no grounds for assuming that two patients have identical cognitive deficits. Clinical classifications such as Wernicke's aphasia, amnesia, or visual agnosia are made on the basis of vague criteria such as 'poor comprehension', which could result from damage to a variety of different cognitive components. Similarly, lesion localisation does not provide a safe grounds for grouping patients. It is unlikely that two patients would have identical lesion localisations and, even if they did, there appear to be substantial individual differences in functional localisation (Ojemann, 1983).

The above discussion reiterates a position that has been advocated by many researchers. The question at issue here is how normal subjects' data should be regarded with respect to individual variation. Discussions of case study methodology often present the argument that although the averaging of data from brain-damaged patients is not justified, such averaging is warranted for normal subjects. For normal subjects, it is assumed that all have the same cognitive system, although the overall efficiency of the system may differ across subjects. The assumption that normal subjects are all alike and that their data can be safely averaged is the basis for standard methodology that is employed with normal subjects in cognitive research, and in experimental psychology in general. In between-subject designs, subjects are randomly assigned to conditions, and the means for the different conditions are compared against the within-condition variance across subjects. Thus, within-condition variance is treated as error variance, that is, random noise. In within-subject designs, subjects participate in two or more conditions, and the interaction of subjects with conditions is treated as the error variance. This experimental research tradition contrasts directly with that of individual differences research where subjects are assumed to differ in their strengths and weaknesses with respect to different cognitive processes (Cronbach, 1975; Vale and Vale, 1969). These differences in abilities across different cognitive components imply that correlations between performance on different types of cognitive tasks can be computed across subjects. High correlations are expected for tasks that draw on the same cognitive mechanisms whereas lower correlations are expected for tasks that draw on different cognitive mechanisms. These correlations may be subjected to various multivariate procedures such as factor analysis in order to determine the set of mental components thought to determine performance across the set of tasks in question. Such procedures have been common in research on intelligence and personality (e.g. see Cardon, Fulker, DeFries and Plomin, 1992; Goldberg, 1993).[1]

Although no one would be likely to question the notion that individuals differ in various cognitive abilities, such as visual–spatial or verbal abilities, researchers in the experimental tradition do not typically question whether the variability of subjects within conditions or the interaction of subjects with conditions may safely be treated as noise. Typically the issues being addressed by such research relate to the precise functioning of various mechanisms within a cognitive domain such as reading, and the assumption may be that individuals do not differ with respect to the relative accuracy or efficiency of what might be considered sub-components of these specific domains. (For example, individuals might be assumed to differ in their overall reading proficiency, but not in their relative proficiency at orthographic *vs* phonological skills.)

The question of individual variability among normal subjects becomes prominent, however, when using the case study approach to do research with brain-damaged subjects. Often the performance of an individual case or a small set of individual cases is contrasted against the performance of a group of normal subjects. Although the patient's data may differ from the pattern demonstrated in the group means, there may be normal subjects within the group who show the same pattern as the patient. Some researchers have argued that the existence of normal subjects who show the same pattern as the patient calls into question the conclusion that the patient's performance arises from the disruption of some cognitive component of processing. For example, in examining

---

[1] The individual differences approach assumes quantitative variation in the efficiency of different cognitive components among normal subjects, and not that individuals differ qualitatively in the collection of cognitive components which they possess. An implication of this is that individuals are not assumed to have unique cognitive components. The existence of unique components would pose a considerable challenge for investigations of both normal and brain-damaged subjects. It should be noted, however, that even quantitative variation can produce strikingly different patterns of results in performance of particular tasks.

lexical processing one might test whether patients show significant semantic priming in a lexical decision task, that is, faster times to decide that a target word is a word if it is preceded by a semantically related word (e.g. priming for *bread* when preceded by *cake*) (see Neely, 1991, for an overview of semantic priming research). Suppose that on several different tasks, the patient fails to show any evidence of semantic priming. On the average, data for normal subjects show a significant semantic priming effect for all of these tasks. Thus, one might conclude that some type of semantic process has been disrupted in the patient. However, an examination of the individual data for the normal subjects may reveal that some subjects show the same pattern as the patient, that is, no evidence of priming. For example, in a study in our laboratory on the automaticity of semantic priming, Shelton and Martin (1992, Experiment 1) found that in three conditions using different procedures for presenting prime-target pairs, an average of 26.7 out of 40 subjects showed a priming effect for associated pairs (e.g. coffee-cup) in the expected direction, obviously implying that an average of 13.3 out of 40 subjects showed a zero or negative priming effect. Given the variability that exists among normal subjects, the question naturally arises as to whether an absence of priming for a patient justifies the conclusion of a semantic deficit.

One simple explanation for the discrepant findings for some normal subjects would be that the atypical pattern for some normal subjects does arise from noise – perhaps the subjects happened not to be paying attention on some critical trials. If this is the explanation, then repeated testing of the same normal subjects under more closely monitored and more motivating conditions should give rise to each subject showing the same pattern as is evident in the group means. Researchers might typically assume that random noise is the source, without carrying out any further tests, and feel that a deficit has been adequately demonstrated if the patient's effect is more than 2 standard deviations below the mean for normal subjects. If random noise is the source of the discrepant data, and all normal subjects do, in fact, show the same pattern when tested more thoroughly, then clearly there is no problem in arguing that an unusual pattern demonstrated by a brain-damaged patient suggests damage to one or more cognitive mechanisms. However, one would have to be sure that the patient had been tested thoroughly enough to warrant the conclusion that his or her pattern could not also be attributed to random noise. Typically, case studies of brain-damaged patients are quite extensive and include many converging operations, thus minimising the likelihood that the patient's pattern could be attributed to noise. Suppose, however, that repeated testing of normal subjects showing an atypical pattern does not solve the problem – different groups of normal subjects show different patterns, with a minority showing a pattern like that of the patient. Several explanations may be possible. One explanation is that some normal subjects also have 'deficits' in certain components of the cognitive system that characterises the majority of normal individuals. That is, there may be individual differences within a cognitive domain with individuals showing a profile of strengths and weaknesses similar to the patterns of dissociations demonstrated in brain-damaged patients, though with the patients typically showing an exaggeration of these patterns. If so, then the results from the normal subjects are perfectly compatible with general assumptions of the cognitive neuropsychological research, in which performance on any given task is assumed to be determined by the functioning of several different components, any of which may be subject to brain damage. For normal subjects, variability in these components may be due to either innate or experiential factors. For the patients, striking deficits in the functioning of particular components result from the brain damage. To make these suggestions more concrete, consider the case of verbal short-term memory. Several patients have been reported in the literature who have very reduced memory span and show a pattern of performance across span tasks indicating a deficit specifically in the retention of phonological information (see Shallice and Vallar, 1990, for an overview). They show no word length effects with auditory or visual presentation, show no phonological similarity effect with visual presentation (though they may show one with auditory presentation), perform better with visual than auditory presentation (the reverse of the normal pattern), and show a reduced or absent recency effect. Such a pattern has been interpreted within various models of short-term memory as demonstrating a specific deficit in the retention of phonological information (Campbell and Butterworth, 1985; Martin, 1993; Vallar and Baddeley, 1984). A phonological retention deficit should lead to particularly impaired performance on nonword repetition, and this has been found to be the case for patient EA (Martin, 1993) and for NC (Martin and Saffran, 1992). In recent years, a few cases have been reported of normal individuals who perform similarly. That is, these individuals report no history of brain injury or neurological disorders, yet show a pattern like that reported by these patients (Baddeley, 1993; Baddeley and Wilson, 1993). In these examples, it seems unlikely that the deficits resulted from any lack of appropriate experiences – all have been exposed to language in a normal fashion throughout their lives. Thus, there is likely to be some deficiency related to phonological storage that is due to innate variability (or perhaps to some minor brain injury whose effects were undetected in everyday activities).

We have recently investigated an individual (WS) in our laboratory who showed this pattern to some degree (Hanten and Martin, 1995), that is, a phonological storage deficit in an individual with no history of neurological disorder. WS is a 28-year-old man who recently obtained a

PhD in biochemistry. Given his academic achievement, it is evident he did not experience any general cognitive deficits. WS came to our attention because the co-workers in his laboratory complained that he often made errors in taking phone messages, misrecording either the name or phone number of the caller, or both. Memory span testing suggested a deficit in phonological retention for WS. Like the patients argued to have a phonological retention deficit, WS performs better with visual than auditory presentation on memory span tasks. On nonword repetition he is below the range for control subjects even for two-item lists, being able to repeat only 50% of lists of two one-syllable nonwords. His word repetition span is about 3-4 items, which is at the low end of the control range (though clearly better than that of some patients with phonological retention deficits who can repeat only one- to two-item word lists). WS shows a phonological similarity effect for both auditory and visual presentation, but his word length effect is small and non-significant. For WS it appears that his phonological retention capacity is restricted, giving rise to some, but not all, of the features of the memory span performance of patients argued to have a phonological retention deficit. Presumably, the phonological storage capacity that he does have is sufficient to give rise to the phonological similarity effect.

Like the cases reported by Baddeley and colleagues, the pattern for WS suggests that there can be striking differences in phonological storage capacity among normal subjects. Thus, the existence of a few normal subjects who show a pattern like that of the patient – though most likely in a less dramatic form – would not appear problematic for concluding that the patient demonstrates a deficit. That is, there would seem to be no logical difficulty in assuming that some individuals with no known brain damage also are relatively deficient in some component of processing. In fact, such variability might be expected to the extent that the different components are independent and subserved by different brain mechanisms.[2]

Another possible source of differences in patterns of performance across normal subjects is that different subjects might adopt different strategies for performing a task. That is, for some unspecified reason, some subjects choose to perform the task using different procedures or criteria than those typically adopted. If so, then the performance displayed by a brain-damaged patient, which diverges from the norm but resembles that of some normal subjects, might be attributed to the patient adopting a strategy similar to that of these atypical normal subjects (see Sala, Logie, Marchetti and Wynn, 1991, for discussion). If this line of reasoning is correct, then the conclusion that the patients' performance results from a disruption of some cognitive component

---

[2] For example, see Kosslyn, Brunn, Cave, and Wallach, 1985, for an examination of the components of a model of mental imagery by using individual differences among normal subjects, and Farah, 1985, for an application of this model to the study of brain-damaged patients.

would seem to be in doubt. Whether this reasoning is sound would seem to depend on the nature of the processing domain under question, specifically with regard to the plausibility of strategies being involved, and whether there is any substantive evidence for strategic effects. There is also the question of why the normal subjects with an aberrant pattern chose an atypical strategy. They may have done so precisely because of their deficiencies in the cognitive components employed by most subjects in performing the task.

For some tasks used in cognitive research evidence does exist for the involvement of different strategies. Returning to the example of semantic priming in the lexical decision task, some researchers have hypothesised that subjects may employ two strategies termed 'expectancy generation' (in which the subject is assumed to generate related words upon seeing a prime) and 'retrospective prime checking' (where the subject is assumed to check whether the target is related to the prime before making a decision about lexicality). Various manipulations of materials (such as changes in the proportion of related word pairs or the time delay between prime and target) have been shown to be related to the likelihood of the involvement of these strategic processes (see Neely (1991), Shelton and Martin (1992) for discussion). Although research has not addressed whether individuals vary in the tendency to use these strategies, it would not seem too unlikely that such differences would be found. The use of these strategies appears to result in larger semantic priming effects than those obtained under conditions in which, presumably, non-strategic, spreading activation is the source of priming (Shelton and Martin, 1992; Tweedy, Lapinski and Schvaneveldt, 1977). This fact, together with the inherent variability in reaction time measures, may lead to some normal subjects showing small or non-existent priming effects because they fail to adopt these strategies. A similar lack of priming for an individual patient might also be plausibly attributed to a failure to adopt these strategies. However, if the researcher is concerned with whether a particular patient does show any evidence of automatic spreading activation, the situation would not appear to be hopeless. Experimental conditions can be chosen that minimise the likelihood that subjects will adopt these strategies (e.g. using a small proportion of related trials and an absence of obvious prime-target pairings). A sufficiently large number of trials could be used making the procedure powerful enough to detect small effects at the single subject level.

In addition, if a patient's failure to show a semantic priming effect does result from an absence of spreading activation, such a deficit would presumably be related to other aspects of the patients' language performance. That is, the issue of whether the patients would or would not show priming most likely arose because of some other aspect of their behaviour such as peculiarities in object naming (Blaxton and Bookheimer, 1993) or dysfluencies in sentence production (Milberg,

Blumstein and Dworetzky, 1987). To the extent that the constellation of symptoms is thought to derive from a single underlying source (e.g. no spreading activation in lexical decision and a particular pattern of word-finding difficulties), patients who show one symptom ought to show the other as well, and patients who show priming ought not to show the same word-finding problems. Thus, there would be a replication of the results across subjects, rendering less plausible the suggestion that the lack of priming was due to a peculiar strategy adopted by an individual patient who otherwise would have shown a typical normal pattern.

In the case of lexical decision there is a large body of data on normal subjects which allows one to determine what kinds of experimental conditions are likely to lead to what types of strategic effects. For many tasks adopted by cognitive neuropsychologists, such a body of evidence may be lacking. Tasks may be made up on the fly because of questions that arise in the testing of patients who show a particularly interesting and unexpected pattern of symptoms. However, what is often of interest is that one patient performs extremely poorly on some tasks but very well on others whereas some other patient may show the reverse pattern on the same tasks. Often there are no normal subjects who show the extreme dissociations demonstrated by the patients. Under these conditions, it would seem unlikely that the results would be due to strategies. To cite a well-known example, one patient may read regular words and nonwords very well, but perform poorly on irregular words, whereas another may read regular and irregular words well, but read nonwords at a very poor level (see Ellis and Young, 1988; Shallice, 1988). It would seem difficult to account for these dissociations on the basis of strategies. That is, why would a subject adopt a strategy that prevented their being able to read nonwords or irregular words if the failure to use this strategy would result in success in reading these items? Certain processing patterns might be evident in the patients' attempts at reading the items which cause them difficulty. For example, the patient with difficulty reading nonwords might produce visually similar words, or the patient with difficulty reading irregular words might produce regularisations. While such processing patterns might be termed 'strategies', these strategies are most likely invoked because the normal mechanisms involved in reading these items have been damaged. To the extent that the term 'strategy' implies a conscious choice (and, therefore, an optional process), the term would seem to be inappropriate when referring to patients who must necessarily rely on certain processes because others have been weakened or rendered inoperative due to brain damage.

Although, in many cases, normal subjects may not show the pattern of performance shown by patients when testing under the same testing conditions (e.g., reading words or judging sentence acceptability under untimed conditions), it is possible that they might show patterns similar to the patients if processing were made difficult in some fashion. For example, suppose that the task is naming written words and nonwords, and low frequency relatively unfamilar words are used and a short response deadline is imposed. It is possible that under these conditions some normal subjects might be induced to make a relatively large number of regularization errors on the irregular words. It is also possible that some other subjects would read the words at a high level but have difficulty reading the nonwords (though showing no such difficulty without a response deadline). Other subjects might perform well with all materials whereas others might perform poorly with all materials. The researcher with these data might then claim to have reproduced in normal subjects some dyslexia syndromes by putting a general strain on the processing system (that is, by using unfamiliar items and imposing a response deadline). This strain has led different subjects to adopt different strategies to deal with the task difficulty. The researcher might then go on to argue that similar constellations of symptoms in brain-damaged patients do not derive from specific deficits but rather to general stress brought on by brain damage, and the selection of different reading strategies on the part of different patients. (Arguments along these lines have recently been put forward in the sentence processing domain – see discussion below.) Of course, this line of reasoning begs the question of what these different reading strategies are and why different subjects should adopt different ones. According to a dual-route model of reading, the normal subjects who under speed stress make errors on irregular words could be said to be using a sublexical sounding-out procedure for reading, whereas the subjects who make errors on nonword reading could be said to be using a lexical procedure. Subjects might show one or the other of these patterns because of the relative strengths of these two routes. That is, as argued earlier, normal subjects could show individual differences in the efficiency of the operation of cognitive components that underlie these two routes. (See Baron and Strawson, 1976, for evidence of individual differences in the efficiency of sublexical and lexical reading routes.) Under speed stress, subjects whose sublexical route operates relatively quickly might produce a response from this route despite accumulating evidence from the lexical route that the input is a real word with an irregular pronunciation. Subjects whose lexical route operates quickly might only have an output from this route at the response deadline, and thus would perform well on word trials but make errors on nonword trials. The performance of subjects who do uniformly well or poorly could result from both routes either operating more quickly or more slowly than average.

Thus, the suggestion that differences in strategies account for different patterns of performance for normal subjects would seem to require further substantiation, whether these different patterns are observed under usual or unusual testing conditions. The use of the term strategy implies that the subjects could perform otherwise. As argued above with respect to the example of reading words under a response deadline – it is possible that the different patterns of performance reflect individual differences in the accuracy or efficiency of the operation of different cognitive components, and that the subject has no option but to perform in the fashion demonstrated. For some experimental tasks, it is possible, though, that there are optional procedures that subjects may invoke which can be controlled by experimental manipulations (as in the example of semantic priming in lexical decision; see also Monsell, Patterson, Hughes, Graham and Milroy, 1992). If so, then it would be incumbent on the experimenter to choose those experimental conditions likely to minimise the engagement of these optional strategies. Whether differences among normal subjects reflect differences in strategies or differences in inherent strengths and weaknesses, it seems that in many experimental paradigms greater information is needed about how normal subjects perform various tasks, particularly with respect to the source of individual differences. The claim that a patient's pattern of performance could be attributed to the adoption of a particular strategy would also seem to require clear evidence with regard to what the strategy is and evidence of its optional nature. For example, suppose that an aphasic patient performed poorly and failed to show a phonological similarity effect on memory span tasks, and the conclusion was drawn that this pattern suggested a deficit in phonological retention. Someone might suggest this result occurred because the patient chose, for some reason, to rely on visual or semantic codes for performing the task, which were not as efficient for performing serial recall. Evidence for this conclusion would have to be demonstrated, for example by showing visual or semantic confusions rather than phonological confusions in recall. The implication that the patient would show a normal level of recall and evidence of phonological coding if induced to do so could be demonstrated by using materials that had different phonological but identical visual representations (e.g. nought – zero – zero – nought – nought (Campbell and Butterworth, 1985)) or materials without a semantic representation (i.e. nonwords). If the patient demonstrated phonological similarity effects and a normal level of recall for these materials, this would constitute solid evidence that the previous results derived from the adoption of a counter-productive strategy. If phonological similarity effects were demonstrated, but performance remained at a poor level, this would suggest that the patient had a decreased ability to retain phonological information, and that the adoption of visual or semantic coding was most likely a response to this deficiency. In general, while it is easy to claim that any differences among normal subjects and differences between a patient and the standard normal pattern reflect 'strategies', it is much more complicated to demonstrate that such is the case. However, such a demonstration would seem to be imperative if these claims are to be taken seriously. Moreover, even when variation in patterns can be attributed to the adoption of optional strategies, experimental manipulations can be undertaken to minimise the involvement of these strategies.

## Sentence processing: normal variation and implications for the understanding of patient deficits

The relevance of individual variation among normal subjects to cognitive neuropsychology has become a central issue in some current debates about sentence processing and sentence processing deficits. Recently, some researchers have argued against the idea that aphasic patients have selective disruptions to various aspects of the semantic and syntactic processes involved in sentence processing. Instead, varying degrees of deficits in working memory or in the use of all types of cues for sentence comprehension have been postulated (Blackwell and Bates, 1995; Miyake, Carpenter and Just, 1994; Wulfeck, Bates and Capasso, 1991). Part of the argument sustaining these views are findings showing that sentences vary in difficulty for normal subjects and that when comprehension processes are stressed in some fashion, different groups of normal subjects show different patterns of performance across sentence types. Before dealing with the specifics of these claims, some general background on the neuropsychology of sentence processing is presented in order to put these claims in perspective. The domain of sentence processing seems to be one of the areas of most contention in the neuropsychological literature. Part of this contentiousness seems to have been inherited from the acrimonious debates between Chomskyan and non-Chomskyan linguists. According to a Chomskyan view, there is a language organ in the brain whose function is to control the acquisition and use of syntax in language production and comprehension (Chomsky, 1980; see Pinker, 1994, for discussion). Non-Chomskyans are vexed by the emphasis on syntax and argue that the purpose of language is to communicate meaning (e.g. Lakoff and Ross, 1976). Syntactic rules, to the extent that such exist, are thought to be tied to properties of lexical items and to serve to express various types of semantic relations (Bresnan, 1981). Consequently, there may be no area of the brain specifically devoted to syntactic processing. Psycholinguists with a Chomskyan bent are likely to prefer modular, rule-based models of sentence processing (e.g. Frazier, 1987) whereas non-Chomskyans are likely to prefer interactive, connectionist models (e.g. MacWhinney, 1991).

An early study of aphasic patients' sentence processing, which attracted enormous interest, seemed to provide support for the Chomskyan view. Caramazza and Zurif (1976) showed that Broca's aphasics (and conduction aphasics) appeared to have a specific deficit in sentence comprehension when comprehension depended on understanding the syntactic structure of the sentence. When given a sentence such as 'The lion that the tiger chased was yellow', these patients had difficulty selecting from a picture showing a lion chasing a tiger and a tiger chasing a lion. (They did not have difficulty, however, if the incorrect picture substituted a different lexical item.) Berndt and Caramazza (1980) expanded on the claims of Caramazza and Zurif (1976) to argue that both the sentence production and sentence comprehension deficits of Broca's aphasics could be attributed to a syntactic deficit. Some patients classed as Broca's aphasics display what is termed agrammatic speech, that is, speech which shows reduced grammatical structure and which is characterised by the omission of function words and grammatical inflections. The positions exemplified by Caramazza and Zurif (1976) and Berndt and Caramazza (1980) were consistent with the notion of a syntactic module localised in the brain which could be selectively disrupted by brain damage.

Evidence against this view began to accumulate, however. Linebarger, Schwartz and Saffran (1983) demonstrated that the Broca's aphasics they tested performed poorly on sentence–picture matching tasks like those employed by Caramazza and Zurif (1976) but nonetheless performed well on grammaticality judgements testing a variety of grammatical structures. Other studies demonstrated dissociations between the agrammatism of speech production of Broca's aphasics and syntactic comprehension, with some patients showing sentence–picture matching performance like that shown by Broca's aphasics yet not showing agrammatic speech (Martin and Blossom-Stach, 1986) and others showing agrammatic speech but no deficit in comprehension (Miceli, Mazzucchi, Menn and Goodglass, 1983).

Despite these findings, some researchers have argued that at least some subset of Broca's aphasics do demonstrate a specific syntactic deficit, though one restricted to particular syntactic rules that have to do with the analysis of arguments that appear in non-standard positions in the sentence (i.e. so-called moved arguments of passives and some relative clause constructions) (Grodzinsky, 1986). Others have argued that these patients do not have specific deficits in syntactic processing, but instead have difficulty in the mapping between grammatical roles and thematic roles (for example, difficulty in mapping subject onto recipient for the verb 'receive') (Saffran and Schwartz, 1988). More recently, others have argued that patients do not have specific deficits in any particular aspect of sentence processing, but instead have a generalised deficit in using all the cues that normal subjects might use in understanding a sentence, perhaps due to general processing capacity restrictions (Blackwell and Bates, 1995). A related view is that aphasic patients in general (not just Broca's aphasics) do not have a deficit in any sentence processing mechanisms per se, but have a deficit in the working memory capacity involved in sentence comprehension (Miyake, Carpenter and Just, 1994). As can be seen from this brief overview, the investigation of sentence processing deficits has been dominated by the group study approach rather than a case study approach by researchers on all sides of the argument with respect to syntactic vs. non-syntactic deficits and specific vs. general deficits. That is, most researchers have focused on agrammatic Broca's aphasics, both because these patients are thought to have preserved lexical-semantic knowledge and because of the apparent grammatical deficits in their speech production. What is missing from this research, for the most part, is a cognitive analysis of sentence processing like that employed in other areas of cognitive neuropsychology. Of course, the issues are quite complex, and explicit models of all the procedures and representations that are involved in production and comprehension are not readily available from the normal literature. (It should be noted that there seems to have been greater development in processing models of speech production, even though experimental data would seem to be more difficult to collect for production than comprehension. See, for example, Dell, 1986, Levelt, 1989.) Relative to studies of language processing at the single word level, little has been done in the way of carrying out case studies of patients showing contrasting deficits in hypothesised components of the comprehension system as a way of testing current models of sentence processing. (Some studies have, however, taken a case study approach. See, for example, Caplan and Futter, 1986; Caplan and Hildebrandt, 1988; Tyler, 1992; Zingeser and Berndt, 1990.)

For those researchers arguing for generalised deficits in sentence processing or deficits in working memory as explanations for sentence comprehension deficits in aphasic patients, the tack taken is often that described earlier, specifically, that of showing that normal subjects under some conditions can be shown to produce data like that shown by some patients (Blackwell and Bates, 1995; Miyake et al., 1994). Researchers taking these positions typically endorse interactive models of sentence processing and object to modular views. Thus, they are motivated to find some means of discounting apparent dissociations in performance across patients which may suggest disruption of different independent components. These researchers argue that since normal subjects can show deficits in processing under some conditions that may mimic the performance of certain patients, it is therefore unnecessary to assume that patients showing different patterns of disruption have deficits in different components of sentence processing.

Research along these lines has been carried out by Bates and colleagues (Wulfeck and Bates, 1991; Wulfeck, Bates and Capasso, 1991; Blackwell and Bates, 1995). In a task in which normal subjects were asked to semantically interpret ungrammatical sentences ('Are kicking the cow the pencils') Bates et al. found that English-speaking subjects relied almost exclusively on word order whereas Italian-speaking subjects made more use of morphology (i.e. noun-verb number agreement) in determining who (or what) was the actor. Wulfeck et al. (1991) demonstrated that on a grammaticality judgement task, English-speaking Broca's aphasics were more accurate in detecting word order violations than agreement errors. Italian-speaking Broca's aphasics showed the same pattern but were worse than the English-speaking aphasics on word order violations and better than them on agreement errors. Wulfeck et al. (1991) attributed these group differences to the lesser importance of word order and greater importance of morphology in Italian than English. For both language groups, the decrements in performance relative to controls were attributed to a general capacity restriction that caused greater deficits for more difficult constructions.

In an attempt to bolster the claims of a capacity restriction as the source of the patients' deficits, Blackwell and Bates (1995) examined normal subjects on a grammaticality judgement task employing word order, word omission, and agreement errors in the incorrect sentences. Subjects performed the task under different levels of a simultaneous digit load, under the assumption that the simultaneous retention of digits would restrict subjects' capacity for sentence analysis. Although normal subjects' performance remained quite high with even a six-item digit load (~96% correct), the error data showed main effects of type of grammatical error and of digit load. With regard to type of grammatical error, sensitivity was best with word order errors, next best with omission errors and worst with agreement errors. The failure to find an interaction between digit load and error type would seem to argue against the two tasks drawing on the same working memory capacity. Nonetheless, the fact that performance was worse with agreement errors than transposition errors, even in the no-load condition, suggests that these errors are generally more difficult to detect, which may account for the pattern seen in the aphasic data. Also, the fact that normal subjects' performance was worse for both types with a digit load suggests that non-specific factors could generally reduce performance on grammaticality judgements, and, thus, such non-specific factors could account for aphasic patients' deficits. Blackwell and Bates go on to argue that the difficulties encountered by Broca's aphasic patients with inflectional morphology in production could also be attributed to a general capacity deficit.

A number of criticisms could be lodged against this research, some of which relate to issues other than the question of individual differences being considered here. At least part of the argument of Bates and colleagues rests, however, on the individual differences between English and Italian-speaking normal subjects and the corresponding difference noted in Broca's aphasics from the two language groups. Whether the differences between the two normal groups result from different weightings of cue types in the two languages is open to debate, since the differing patterns were obtained in subjects' attempts to understand ungrammatical sentences. The differential use of cues may have resulted because of strategies the subjects invoked to handle these unusual 'sentences'. Assume, however, that in sentence processing, normal Italian and English subjects do make differential use of different types of cues in arriving at a semantic interpretation of a sentence. Thus, in English, the output of processes relating sentence position (i.e. word order) to grammatical role may have greater weight than the output of processes detecting subject–verb agreement. In a connectionist type model, one might assume greater connection strengths from inputs due to word order. In Italian, the relative strengths could be reversed. Generalised brain damage across connections might serve to exaggerate this pattern of differential weights. However, such evidence would not demonstrate that no distinction or localisability was possible for the connections subserving word order and those subserving morphology. The question would be are there patients who do not show an exaggeration of the normal pattern, but who show the reverse? That is, among English-speaking aphasics, are there those who show difficulties with word order but not with morphology? The answer seems to be yes, but only with respect to a particular aspect of word order. For example, Martin and Blossom-Stach (1986) reported a mild Wernicke's aphasic patient who produced and understood morphology correctly, but yet had difficulty in assigning agent and object in simple transitive sentences, both in comprehension and production. A similar case was reported by Caramazza and Miceli (1991). It should be noted that neither patient had any difficulty with word order in terms of knowing what sequences of word classes are allowable. Rather, their comprehension problem had to do with some step in the process that links position in the sentence to grammatical role and that links grammatical role to thematic role.

Miyake, Carpenter and Just (1994) have adopted a theoretical viewpoint similar to that of Bates and colleagues with regard to the nature of comprehension deficits in aphasic patients, though their claims seem to be more sweeping. These researchers have adopted an individual differences approach in their analysis of normal subjects' performance. Just and Carpenter (1992) presented a theoretical analysis of normal subjects in which they argued that normal individuals differ in their working memory capacity for sentence processing, and these differences have a number of consequences for comprehension patterns. Typically, the difference in performance between high and low capacity subjects increases as sentence difficulty increases. For example, identifying the referent of a pronoun can be carried out equally well by high and low capacity subjects if the referent is near the pronoun in the sentence whereas an advantage for high capacity subjects is obtained when the referent is farther away (Daneman and Carpenter, 1980). In one study MacDonald, Just and Carpenter (1992) demonstrated a deficit in comprehension for high span subjects on syntactically ambiguous sentences when the simpler interpretation of the ambiguity proved correct. They interpreted this finding as resulting from the high capacity subjects' being able to maintain both the simpler and more complex interpretations simultaneously whereas the low capacity subjects could only maintain the simpler interpretation. When the simpler interpretation proved correct, the high capacity subjects were at a disadvantage because they had to suppress the more complex interpretation. Miyake et al. (1994) have suggested that aphasic subjects' comprehension deficits result from their having even greater restrictions in capacity than the low capacity normal subjects. That is, they are hypothesised to be simply farther down on the capacity scale. In support of this contention they discuss evidence in the literature indicating that on sentence comprehension measures, aphasic patients from various clinical groups (e.g. Broca's, Wernicke's, conduction) show the same decline in performance with increasing structural complexity, but with the effect of complexity increasing as the patient groups' overall degree of deficit increases. The experiments carried out by Miyake et al. examined normal subjects' comprehension of similar sentence structures when the sentences were presented using a rapid serial visual presentation paradigm with either 120 or 200 ms per word. They found that normal subjects showed a similar rank ordering of performance in relation to structural complexity as that found for aphasic patients.

As discussed in relation to the findings of Bates and colleagues (e.g. Blackwell and Bates, 1995), one might object that not all aphasic patients show the same pattern of performance across sentence types as that reported in the group means. Miyake et al. (1994), however, analysed the normal subjects' data using a cluster analysis and showed that different patterns of performance across sentence type were found for the different clusters of subjects. They claim that the patterns identified were similar to those reported by Caplan and Hildebrandt (1988), who performed a cluster analysis on aphasic patients' comprehension performance.

A number of objections can be raised with regard to the interpretations of the results of the Miyake et al. study and to the general approach of Just and Carpenter to sentence processing (see Caplan and Waters (in press) and Martin (in press) for discussion). The claim that the normal subgroups replicated the patterns displayed by patients is open to debate. For example, none of the subgroups of normal subjects showed poor performance on simple transitive passive sentences, though clearly some aphasic patients do demonstrate such difficulties. (See Caplan and Waters for a discussion of this and other discrepancies.)

With regard to the central issue here of the implications of normal variation, Miyake et al. (1994) claim that because normal subjects demonstrate different patterns of performance across sentence types, and because these subjects have no brain damage, such differences cannot be attributed to the disruption of different cognitive components. Hence, finding dissociations (and double dissociations) across patients' comprehension patterns does not imply the disruption of independent cognitive components. Although finding the same rank ordering of sentence difficulty for both aphasic patients and normal subjects is consistent with Miyake et al.'s restricted capacity hypothesis, these findings are also consistent with accounts that assume that performance decrements derive from the malfunctioning of various components underlying comprehension. As argued by Martin (in press), more difficult sentences would presumably engage more cognitive components. Assuming that brain damage randomly affected these components, the more components that are involved, the more likely that at least one of them has been affected, with the consequence that comprehension will fail. For normal subjects, one might assume that for rapid presentation, it is possible that one or more of the processes involved in integrating the current word with the ongoing interpretation of the sentence might not be completed before the next word has to be dealt with. With more difficult sentences, more processes would typically be involved, increasing the probability of a failure to complete these processes.

The findings of subgroups of normal subjects showing comprehension patterns allegedly like those demonstrated by different patient groups might seem more damaging to the claim of a disruption of independent components in the patients. However, along the lines argued earlier, one might hypothesise that normal subjects have strengths and weaknesses in various aspects of sentence processing, and that their performance under conditions that stress processing speed results from the failure of some of the weaker components to complete their processing quickly enough. Under these conditions, subjects' responses are dependent on those components that have completed processing. For example, suppose that for some subjects, the processes involved in mapping between grammatical and thematic roles cannot be carried out quickly enough when sentences are presented in a rapid serial visual presentation format. The result may be that these subjects fall back on heuristic processes that also influence comprehension under more normal sentence processing conditions, such as heuristics relating thematic role to position in the sentence (e.g. the first noun before the verb is likely to be the agent, etc.) (Caplan, Hildebrandt and Waters, 1994; Huttenlocher, Eisenberg and Strauss, 1968). This pattern of using word order for thematic role assignment has been noted in some aphasic patients (Caplan and Futter, 1986).

Thus, the assumption of the involvement of independent components could be used to account for both patient and normal subjects' performance. It is not entirely clear how Miyake et al. (1994) account for the differences observed between different groups of subjects. They suggest that noise or strategic effects might account for differences among subjects. The same considerations raised earlier with regard to these two explanations apply here as well. The issue of noise could be assessed by repeated testing. To assess whether strategies were involved, some specific suggestions would be needed with regard to what these strategies might be. Then testing could be carried out under conditions designed to prevent the involvement of these strategies. Somewhat curiously, Miyake et al. also suggest that differences between normal subjects might be due to differences in the relative efficiency of different processes. This possibility is identical to the suggestion presented here that normal subjects show different strengths and weaknesses in the component processes involved in sentence comprehension. Furthermore, if Miyake et al. are willing to make this assumption, there would seem to be no need to make the further assumption of individual differences in working memory capacity.

With regard to attributing variations in patients' performance to noise or strategic effects, existing patient data would seem to be difficult to accommodate by such explanations. As noted in Martin (in press), some patients perform at a high level on some types of difficult constructions such as centre-embedded relative clause sentences but perform near chance on others, such as so-called 'raising' constructions (e.g. 'John seemed to a friend of Bill's to be shaving'), whereas other patients show the reverse (Caplan and Hildebrandt, 1988). It is hard to imagine what kind of strategies could be employed to give rise to these contrasting patterns. Without some suggestion of what these strategies might be and some empirical evidence for the employment of such strategies, it is difficult to take the claims of Miyake et al. seriously.

## Conclusions

Individual differences among normal subjects have been shown to exist in various cognitive domains, and are likely to be ubiquitous. Such differences are typically ignored by researchers, both those who carry out experimental research with normal subjects and those who use the data from normal subjects as a standard against which to compare the performance of neuropsychological cases. Some recent theorising in neuropsychology has pointed to the differences among normal subjects as invalidating claims that contrasting patterns in the performance of different brain-damaged patients indicate impairments to different cognitive components. However, rather than contradicting the claims of separable components, variations in performance among normal subjects may support these claims by revealing different strengths and weaknesses among normal subjects in these components.

It seems clear, however, that more needs to be known about the source of individual differences among normal subjects. For most expermental studies, even the number of subjects showing an effect in a particular direction is usually not reported. Even less often is there any information provided about the stability of patterns across repeated testing. A few studies have demonstrated the importance of looking at individual variation in normal subjects in studies examining performance in specific cognitive domains. For example, Martin and Caramazza (1980), in a study of category learning, showed that the overall mean data seemed to support a prototype view, with reaction time and accuracy measures of category decisions relating to the similarity of an exemplar to the prototype. However, when subjects' data were analysed individually, it was found that subjects used a sequence of logical feature tests, with different subjects using different features as the basis of these tests. In this study, the group findings reflected none of the individual subjects' patterns. Other studies have demonstrated that even though the mean data represent a majority of the subjects, distinctive subgroups of subjects exist who perform in substantially different fashion. For example, MacLeod, Hunt and Mathews (1978) reported that in a sentence verification paradigm for locative sentences (e.g. 'Plus is above star'), a majority of subjects were well-fit by a linguistic coding model, whereas a smaller group showed evidence of using a spatial strategy.

Paradoxically, some researchers have argued that because averaging of group data is carried out with normal subjects, even though differences exist among these subjects, therefore group studies are warranted with brain-damaged cases (Caplan, 1988). The discussion here is leading to the opposite conclusion. The existence of variation among normal subjects indicates that case studies of normal subjects are called for, as they are for brain-damaged patients. For normal subjects, such studies would more likely be simultaneous studies of many individual cases, rather than the study of a single case often seen in neuropsychology. (The reason for the difference is obvious – normal subjects are not rare.) The presentation of individual data for normal subjects would provide a much clearer picture of the degree of individual variability in effect size (and direction) than is available from current measures such as standard error. It seems likely that open presentation of individual data would lead to attempts to determine the stability of individual patterns. It might also lead to greater attempts to determine whether these different patterns can be eliminated when procedures are employed to discourage various types of strategic processing. For those differences which appear to be inherent to differing cognitive processing abilities across normal subjects, the contrasting patterns may lead to inferences about the nature of the cognitive system, like those that have been derived from neuropsychological studies. It would seem that such data from normal subjects, thoroughly analysed with respect to individual differences, would provide much better grounds for developing theories of the nature of cognition, than conclusions based on group effects, which may not reflect even the majority of normal subjects.

# References

Baddeley, A.D. (1993). Short-term phonological memory and long-term learning: A single case study. *European Journal of Cognitive Psychology*, **5**, 129–148.

Baddeley, A.D. and Wilson, B.A. (1993). A developmental deficit in short-term phonological memory: Implications for language and reading. *Memory*, **1**, 65–78.

Baron, J. and Strawson, C. (1976). Use of orthographic and word-specific knowledge in reading words aloud. *Journal of Experimental Psychology: Human Perception and Performance*, **2**, 386–393.

Berndt, R. and Caramazza, A. (1980). A redefinition of the syndrome of Broca's aphasia: Implications for a neuropsychological theory of language. *Applied Psycholinguistics*, **1**, 225–278.

Blackwell, A. and Bates, E. (1995). Inducing agrammatic profiles in normals: Evidence for the selective vulnerability of morphology under cognitive resource limitation. *Journal of Cognitive Neuroscience*, **7**, 228–257.

Blaxton, T. and Bookheimer, S. (1993). Retrieval inhibition in anomia. *Brain and Language*, **44**, 221–237.

Bresnan, J. (1981). An approach to universal grammar and the mental representation of language. *Cognition*, **10**, 39–52.

Campbell, R. and Butterworth, B. (1985). *Quarterly Journal of Experimental Psychology*, **37**, 435–475.

Caplan, D. (1988). On the role of group studies in neuropsychological and pathopsychological research. *Cognitive Neuropsychology*, **5**, 535–547.

Caplan, D. and Futter, C. (1986). Assignment of nouns to thematic roles in sentence comprehension by an agrammatic patient. *Brain and Language*, **27**, 117–134.

Caplan, D. and Hildebrandt, N. (1988). *Disorders of Syntactic Comprehension*. Cambridge, MA: MIT Press.

Caplan, D. and Waters, G. (in press). Aphasic disorders of syntactic comprehension and working memory. *Cognitive Neuropsychology*.

Caplan, D., Hildebrandt, N. and Waters, G. (1994). Interaction of verb selectional restrictions, noun animacy and syntactic form in sentence processing. *Language and Cognitive Processes*, **9**, 549–585.

Caramazza, A. (1984). The logic of neuropsychological research and the problem of patient classification. *Brain and Language*, **21**, 9–20.

Caramazza, A. and McCloskey, M. (1988). The case for single-patient studies. *Cognitive Neuropsychology*, **5**, 517–528.

Caramazza, A. and Miceli, G. (1991). Selective impairment of thematic role assignment in sentence processing. *Brain and Language*, **41**, 402–436.

Caramazza, A. and Zurif, E. (1976). Dissociation of algorithmic and heuristic processes in language comprehension: Evidence from aphasia. *Brain and Language*, **3**, 572–582.

Cardon, L. R., Fulker, D. W., De Fries, J. C. and Plomin, R. (1992). Multivariate genetic analysis of specific cognitive abilities in the Colorado adoption project at age 7. *Intelligence*, **16**, 383–400.

Chomsky, N. (1980). *Rules and Representations*. New York: Columbia University Press.

Cronbach, L.J. (1975). Beyond the two disciplines of scientific psychology. *American Psychologist*, 30, 116–127.

Daneman, M. and Carpenter, P. (1980). Individual differences in working memory and reading. *Journal of Verbal Learning and Verbal Behaviour*, 19, 450–466.

Dell, G. (1986). A spreading-activation theory of retrieval in sentence production. *Psychological Review*, 93, 283–321.

Ellis, A. and Young, A. (1987). *Human Cognitive Neuropsychology*. London: Erlbaum.

Farah, M. (1985). The neurological basis of mental imagery: A componential analysis. In S. Pinker (Ed.) *Visual Cognition*. Amsterdam: Elsevier.

Frazier, L. (1987). Sentence processing: A tutorial review. In M. Coltheart (Ed.) *Attention and Performance XII: The Psychology of Reading*. Hillsdale, N.J.: Erlbaum.

Goldberg, L.R. (1993). The structure of phenotypic personality traits. *American Psychologist*, 48, 26–34.

Grodzinsky, Y. (1986). Language deficits and the theory of syntax. *Brain and Language*, 27, 135–159.

Hanten, G. and Martin, R.C. (1995). Auditory and phonological short-term memory: *A case study of an individual without neurological disorder*. Unpublished manuscript.

Huttenlocher, J., Eisenberg, K. and Strauss, S. (1968). Comprehension: relation between perceived actor and logical subject. *Journal of Verbal Learning and Verbal Behaviour*, 7, 527–530.

Just, M. and Carpenter, P. (1992). A capacity theory of comprehension: Individual differences in working memory. *Psychological Review*, 99, 122–149.

Kosslyn, S., Brunn, J., Cave, K.R. and Wallach, R.W. (1985). Individual differences in mental imagery ability: A computational analysis. In S.Pinker (Ed.) *Visual Cognition*. Amsterdam: Elsevier.

Lakoff, G. and Ross, J.R. (1976). Is deep structure necessary? In J. McCawley (Ed.) *Syntax and Semantics*, Vol. 7. New York: Academic Press.

Levelt, W.J.M. (1989). *Speaking: From Intention to Articulation*. Cambridge, MA.: MIT Press.

Linebarger, M., Schwartz, M. and Saffran, E. (1983). Sensitivity to grammatical structure in so-called agrammatic aphasics. *Cognition*, 13, 361–392.

MacDonald, M., Just, M. and Carpenter, P. (1992). Working memory constraints and the processing of syntactic ambiguity. *Cognitive Psychology*, 24, 56–98.

MacLeod, C.M., Hunt, E.B. and Mathews, N.N. (1978). Individual differences in the verification of sentence–picture relationships. *Journal of Verbal Learning and Verbal Behaviour*, 17, 493–507.

MacWhinney, B. (1991). Connectionism as a framework for language acquisition. In J. Miller (Ed.) *Research on Child Language Disorders: A Decade of Progress*. Austin, TX.: Pro-Ed.

Martín, N. and Saffran, E.M. (1992). A computational account of deep dysphasia: Evidence from a single case study. *Brain and Language*, 43, 240–274.

Martin, R.C. (1993). Short-term memory and sentence processing: Evidence from neuropsychology. *Memory and Cognition*, 21, 176–183.

Martin, R.C. (in press). Working memory doesn't work: A critique of Miyake et al.'s capacity theory of aphasic comprehension deficits. *Cognitive Neuropsychology*.

Martin, R.C. and Blossom-Stach, C. (1986). Evidence of syntactic deficits in a fluent aphasic. *Brain and Language*, 38, 196–234.

Martin, R. C. and Caramazza, A. (1980). Classification in well-defined and ill-defined categories: Evidence for common processing strategies. *Journal of Experimental Psychology: General*, 109, 320–353.

Miceli, G., Mazzucchi, A., Menn, L. and Goodglass, H. (1983). Contrasting cases of Italian agrammatic aphasia without comprehension disorder. *Brain and Language*, **19**, 65–97.

Milberg, W., Blumstein, S. E. and Dworetzky, B. (1987). Processing of lexical ambiguities in aphasia. *Brain and Language*, **31**, 138–150.

Miyake, A., Carpenter, P. A. and Just, M.A. (1994). A capacity approach to syntactic comprehension disorders: Making normal adults perform like aphasic patients. *Cognitive Neuropsychology*, **11**, 671–717.

Monsell, S., Patterson, K., Hughes, A., Graham, C. and Milroy, R. (1992). Lexical and sublexical translation of spelling to sound: Strategic anticipation of lexical status. *Journal of Experimental Psychology: Learning, Memory and Cognition*, **18**, 452–467.

Neely, J.H. (1991). Semantic priming in visual word recognition: A selective review of current theories and findings. In D. Besner and G. Humphreys (Eds) *Basic Processes in Reading: Visual Word Recognition*, pp. 264–336. Hillsdale, N.J.: Erlbaum.

Ojemann, G. (1983). Brain organisation for language from the perspective of electrical stimulation mapping. *Brain and Behavioural Sciences*, **6**, 189–230.

Pinker, S. (1994). *The Language Instinct*. New York: W. Morrow.

Robertson, L., Knight, R., Rafal, R. and Shimamura, A. (1993). Cognitive neuropsychology is more than single-case studies. *Journal of Experimental Psychology: Learning, Memory and Cognition*, **19**, 710–717.

Saffran, E. and Schwartz, M. (1988). 'Agrammatic' comprehension it's not: Alternatives and implications. *Aphasiology*, **2**, 389–394.

Sala, S.D., Logie, R.H., Marchetti, C. and Wynn, V. (1991). Case studies in working memory: A case for single cases? *Cortex*, **27**, 169–191.

Shallice, T. (1988). *From Neuropsychology to Mental Structure*. New York: Cambridge.

Shallice, T. and Vallar, G. (1990). The impairment of auditory–verbal short-term storage. In G. Vallar and T. Shallice (Eds) *Neurospychological Impairments of Short-term Memory*. New York: Cambridge.

Shelton, J.R. and Martin, R.C. (1992). How semantic is automatic semantic priming? *Journal of Experimental Psychology: Learning, Memory and Cognition*, **18**, 1191–1209.

Tweedy, J.R., Lapinski, R.H. and Schvaneveldt, R.W. (1977). Semantic-context effects on word recognition: Influence of varying the proportion of items presented in an appropriate context. *Memory and Cognition*, **5**, 84–89.

Tyler, L. (1992). *Spoken Language Comprehension: An Experimental Approach to Disordered and Normal Processing*. Cambridge, MA: MIT Press.

Vale, J.R. and Vale, C.A. (1969). Individual differences and general laws in psychology: A reconciliation. *American Psychologist*, **24**, 1093–1108.

Vallar, G. and Baddeley, A.D. (1984). Fractionation of working memory: Neuropsychological evidence for a phonological short-term store. *Journal of Verbal Learning and Verbal Behaviour*, **23**, 121–142.

Warrington, E.K. and Shallice, T. (1969). The selective impairment of auditory-verbal short-term memory. *Brain*, **92**, 885–896.

Wulfeck, B. and Bates, E. (1991). Differential sensitivity to errors of agreement and word order in Broca's aphasia. *Journal of Cognitive Neuroscience*, **3**, 258–272.

Wulfeck, B., Bates, E. and Capasso, R. (1991). A cross-linguistic study of grammaticality judgments in Broca's aphasia. *Brain and Language*, **41**, 311–336.

Zingeser, L. and Berndt, R.S. (1990). Retrieval of nouns and verbs in agrammatism and anomia. *Brain and Language*, **39**, 14–32.

# Chapter 6
# Symptoms of Disorder without Impairment: The Written and Spoken Errors of Bilinguals

BARBARA J. DODD, LYDIA K.H. SO AND LI WEI

## Abstract

*Assumptions about the nature of normal language function based on monolingual language acquisition and its disorders may lead to an incomplete understanding of language processing. Two experiments assessed normal subjects with bilingual language learning experience. The first experiment describes Hong Kong university students, with high levels of literacy in both Chinese and English, who performed poorly on tasks assessing phonological awareness. Phonological awareness has been shown to be closely associated with alphabetic literacy. These students' first written language was Chinese, learned as logographs. The second experiment shows that young bilingual children's acquisition of phonology is characterised by unusual error patterns in both languages. Some of these error patterns are indicative of phonological disorder in monolingual children. The results of both experiments suggest that particular language learning experience can lead to language behaviour in normal people that mimics that associated with impairment.*

## Introduction

Much of my early research into phonological acquisition was based on the assumption that it was possible to better understand the nature of normal function by describing the effects of specific types of impairment, where impairment is a disturbance of structure or function at the organ level, whether psychological, physiological or anatomical (WHO, 1980). To that end I described the phonological systems and abilities of children who were profoundly hearing impaired in order to evaluate the contribution of audition. Similarly, I investigated groups of children with different types of cognitive impairment to assess how such impairments

119

would affect phonological development. Some of those experiments have been repeated by other researchers and sometimes conflicting findings have been reported. I then searched the method sections for an explanation. The answer often lay with the subject population. They were a different age, had a different language learning experience, or were learning a language other than English. While such explanations are often very plausible they create another problem. If there are large individual differences amongst the population being studied, could it be that the behaviour observed reflects more than just normal development minus the effects of the specific impairment. Another way of putting it is, to what extent does the observed behaviour of an individual reflect the type of impairment?[1] Obviously, this is a difficult question to answer. However, two recent experiments, one done with Lydia So and the other with Li Wei throw some light on the issue.

## Experiment one

There is now strong evidence that inadequate knowledge and awareness of the sound structure of language, due to phonological processing deficits, constrains the acquisition of literacy skills. Many children with specific reading disability have a deficit that limits the ability to decode text using grapheme–phoneme conversion rules (Rack, Snowling and Olsen, 1992). Further, as might be predicted, Dodd et al. (1995) found that on standard tests of reading and spelling, children with a spoken phonological disorder performed more poorly than matched controls or children with delayed phonological development. Both these groups of children, those with specific reading disability and those with a spoken phonological disorder, also often perform poorly on tests of phonological awareness such as segmentation, creation of Spoonerisms, sound deletion and rhyming (Dodd, Leahy and Hambly, 1989; Leitao, Hogben and Fletcher, 1995; Gillon and Dodd, 1994). Such findings lead to the conclusion that an impairment in phonological processing is associated with the difficulties many children have in learning to read and spell.

One question raised by these findings concerns whether it is possible to acquire adequate literacy skills in the absence of phonological coding ability. There are a number of cases reported in the literature. For example, RE, Campbell and Butterworth's (1985) case, was able to read real words despite performing very poorly on tasks of phonological awareness and nonword reading. They concluded that RE had learned to read and spell using a direct visual route. Nevertheless, such cases appear to be rare. So my experience when I was external examiner at Hong Kong University, where the medium of instruction is English, was surprising. Despite being trained in phonetics, the speech pathology students' performance indicated that many of them had very poor phonemic

---

[1] See Martin, this volume, for consideration of this question in the light of acquired disorders.

segmentation skills. For example, when designing sets of minimally paired stimuli to elicit the /k/ – /t/ distinction ([kæp] *vs* [tæp]) some students would include as /t/-words those with initial /θ/ ([θɪk] *vs* [kɪk]), indicating that their choice was based on how words looked (thick, kick) when written down rather than how they sounded. Further, while these students' written exam papers contained semantic and syntactic errors, they rarely made spelling errors. These observations prompted the following experiment which investigated the phonological coding abilities of three groups of university students whose first spoken language was Cantonese but who had also learned English as a spoken and written language.

# Method

## Subjects

Three groups of 20 undergraduate subjects (27 males and 33 females) with a mean age of 21 years participated in the study. The groups were selected on the basis of their first language literacy acquisition process and tertiary language experience. All subjects' first spoken language was Cantonese and they had completed at least one year of university study. They had no previous spoken language or literacy difficulties in their first language, and the students' level of competence in English as a second language was similar.

*Group 1*: Twenty students, from various departments within Hong Kong University where the language of instruction was English, such as Science and Medicine, volunteered to participate. Their first written language was Chinese learned as logographs, i.e. they had not learned an alphabetic system before they were exposed to English. The approach to reading in Hong Kong is largely 'look and say'. Children are taught character-to-pronunciation mappings, without the mediation of an alphabetic system (Taft and Chen, 1992). English as a second language is usually introduced in the third year of primary school. The 'look and say' process of instruction is also used for learning written English (Huang and Hanley, 1994; Leong, 1973). English teaching was maintained throughout their primary and secondary education, although it was not the general medium of instruction.

*Group 2*: Another 20 Hong Kong University students were tested. These students were from the Department of Speech and Hearing Science where they were studying Speech Pathology and had already completed two years of training in phonetics. Their training in phonetics was the only difference between the two groups of Hong Kong students.

*Group 3:*   Twenty students who were studying English at the Guangzhou
Foreign Language Institute were assessed whose first written
language was Chinese logographs learned using pinyin. In
1958, as part of a general language reform movement, an
alphabetic system employing Latin symbols, called pinyin, was
introduced in mainland China. Pinyin is essentially a phonemic representation of the language in Roman letters (Huang
and Hanley, 1994; Read, Zhang, Nie and Ding, 1986), used to
promote the standard dialect and to facilitate initial learning
of reading the Chinese logographic system (Barnitz, 1978).

## Procedure

The subjects were tested individually in one 60-minute session in a quiet
room at their University. A series of tasks, described below, assessed
phonological awareness, reading and spelling of real and nonwords. All
subjects received the tasks in the same order. Practice items were given
for all tasks.

## Phonological processing tasks

### Syllable segmentation

Subjects listened to 16 words and were required to count the number of
syllables to assess their awareness of sounds at the sublexical level.
There were four items of two-, three-, four- and five-syllable words
presented in random order (e.g. advice, opportunity).

### Onset-rime awareness

This task assessed awareness of sub-syllabic units. Subjects were shown
five sets of five pictures and told to point to the pictures starting with a
particular sound (e.g. 'b' picture set: pear, dog, sun, bed, bottle).

### Rhyme production

This task assessed the ability to generate rhyming words. Subjects were
asked, 'Tell me as many words as you can that rhyme with ...'. There were
ten items (e.g. camp, barge). Up to four rhymes were scored for each
target word.

### Phoneme segmentation

This task required subjects to analyse the internal composition of words
at the phonemic level by counting the number of constituent sounds.
The 24 words, increasing in number of sounds, were presented orally
and included words that were: real words with a one-to-one phoneme-

to-grapheme correspondence (e.g. stamp); real words with a one-to-many phoneme-to-grapheme correspondence (e.g. whistle); nonsense words (e.g. stelp).

## Spoonerisms

This task tapped the subjects' ability to segment words and apply a novel phonological rule (adapted from Perin, 1983). It assessed the subject's ability to manipulate complex phonemic information. The subjects were required to create Spoonerisms of eight word pairs by transposing the initial phonemes of each pair (e.g. big dog → dig bog; soft cheese → choft seese; shark dip → dark ship). The subjects were encouraged to respond to each item.

## Reading tasks

The following tasks assessed reading skills in terms of the strategies used in orthographic decoding.

## Word reading

Subjects were asked to read a list of 24 words of increasing length (e.g. map, bone, biscuit, psychiatry). The list included words that had a one-to-one phoneme-to-grapheme correspondence (e.g. wombat); words where a more complex phoneme-grapheme correspondence rule needed to be known (e.g. liquid); and irregular words (e.g. xylophone).

## Nonword reading

Subjects were asked to read aloud a list of 24 nonwords, 12 of which were phonologically plausible spellings of real words (e.g. wissul) and 12 of which were true nonwords (e.g. framyip).

## Visual rhyme recognition

Subjects were required to decide whether 20 written word pairs rhymed. Four types of word pairs were presented: orthographically similar rhyming words (e.g. ring/sing); orthographically dissimilar rhyming words (e.g. core/raw); orthographically similar non-rhyming words (e.g. worm/form); and orthographically dissimilar non-rhyming words (e.g. rot/rat).

## Spelling tasks

## Real word spelling

Twenty-four real words were presented, twice in isolation and once in a phrase, for writing to dictation. Eight stimulus items could be generated by using direct phoneme–grapheme correspondences (e.g. impedi-ment); eight could be generated by rule knowledge (e.g. cake) and eight were irregular (e.g. aquarium).

## Nonword spelling

Twenty nonwords were presented. Each word was repeated three times. It was emphasised that there was no correct spelling for the nonwords, that the words should be written according to how they sound. Ten of the items could be spelled by analogy to real words (e.g. flecipe)

## Results

Table 6.1 shows the means, standard deviations and results of ANOVAs with Bonferroni-protected *post hoc* tests for the phonological awareness tasks. The results show that Group 1, the Hong Kong students with neither training in phonetics nor pinyin, performed more poorly than the other two groups on all tasks requiring awareness at the sub-syllabic level: onset rime; rhyme generation; phoneme segmentation; Spooner-isms; and identification of visual rhyme. In contrast, Group 2, the Hong Kong speech pathology students who had completed two years training in phonetics, performed more poorly than the Guangzhou students (who had learned written Chinese using pinyin) on only two of these tasks: phoneme segmentation and visual rhyme identification. The only task that elicited poorer performance by the Guangzhou students than the Hong Kong students was the ability to identify the number of sylla-bles in words.

Table 6.2 shows the means and standard deviations for the nonword reading and spelling tasks. A two-factor ANOVA for the real and nonword reading task revealed a significant Groups term ($F$ (2,57) = 28.622, $p < 0.001$), a significant Effect of Word Type ($F$ (1,57) = 164.861, $p < 0.001$) and a significant Interaction ($F$ (2,57) = 30.048, $p < 0.001$). *Post hoc* Bonferroni-protected Newman–Keuls testing between groups showed that while the groups performed equally well when reading real words, nonwords elicited differences between all three groups with Group 1 performing more poorly than Group 2 (Critical Value (CV) = 10.2, Observed Value (OV) = 15.6) and Group 3 (CV = 12.4, OV = 40.9), and Group 3 performing better than Group 2 (CV = 11.6, OV = 25.3). Within-group comparisons showed that while both groups of Hong Kong students were better at reading real words than nonwords (Group 1: CV = 9.9, OV = 37.9, Group 2: CV = 11.1, OV = 30.1), the Guangzhou group performed equally across these two tasks. A two-factor ANOVA for the real and nonword spelling task revealed a significant Groups term ($F$ (2,57) = 4.728, $p < 0.025$), a significant Effect of Word Type ($F$ (1,57) = 248.934, $p < 0.001$) and a significant Interaction ($F$ (2,57) = 8.9,

$p < 0.001$). *Post hoc* Bonferroni-protected Newman–Keuls testing between groups showed that the three groups performed equally well when spelling real words, but that Group 1 performed more poorly than the other two groups when spelling nonwords (Group 2: CV = 11.5, OV = 12.5, Group 3: CV = 13.1, OV = 19.4). Within-group comparisons showed that all three groups performed better when spelling real words than nonwords (Group 1: CV = 10.7, OV = 37.8; Group 2: CV = 11.2, OV = 32.7; Group 3: CV = 9.95, OV = 19.0).

**Table 6.1** Total mean percentage correct (SD) on phonological awareness tasks

| | Mean | SD | Hong Kong 1 | Hong Kong 2 | Guangzhou |
|---|---|---|---|---|---|
| *Total percentage correct on Syllable Segmentation Task ($F_{2,57}=16.001, p < 0.001$)* | | | | | |
| HK 1 | 90.6% | 12.3 | – | NS | * |
| HK 2 | 96.3% | 5.5 | | – | * |
| Guangzhou | 77.2% | 13.4 | | | – |
| *Total correct on Onset Rime Task (Max 10) ($F_{2,57} = 13.994, p < 0.001$)* | | | | | |
| HK 1 | 8.0 | 1.3 | – | * | * |
| HK 2 | 9.4 | 0.9 | | – | NS |
| Guangzhou | 9.6 | 0.5 | | | – |
| *Number of Rhymes Generated (Max = 40) ($F_{2,57} = 10.872, p < 0.001$)* | | | | | |
| HK 1 | 5.0 | 3.2 | – | * | * |
| HK 2 | 8.5 | 4.1 | | – | NS |
| Guangzhou | 10.6 | 4.7 | | | – |
| *Total percentage correct on Phoneme Segmentation Task ($F_{2,57} = 40.480, p < 0.001$)* | | | | | |
| HK 1 | 45.1% | 18.0 | – | * | * |
| HK 2 | 69.7% | 11.7 | | – | * |
| Guangzhou | 82.8% | 9.2 | | | – |
| *Total percentage correct on Spoonerism Creation Task ($F_{2,57} = 11.829, p < 0.001$)* | | | | | |
| HK 1 | 62.3% | 24.0 | – | * | * |
| HK 2 | 84.5% | 14.4 | | – | NS |
| Guangzhou | 86.8% | 12.2 | | | – |
| *Total percentage correct on Visual Rhyme Judgement Task ($F_{2,57} = 19.224, p < 0.001$)* | | | | | |
| HK 1 | 72.0% | 11.5 | – | * | * |
| HK 2 | 82.0% | 8.7 | | – | * |
| Guangzhou | 90.5% | 7.8 | | | – |

* Denotes pairs of groups significantly different at the 0.01 level, Bonferroni-protected.

**Table 6.2** Group means (SD) for reading and spelling tasks

| Task | Group 1 Hong Kong | Group 2 Hong Kong | Group 3 Guangzhou |
|------|------------------|------------------|-------------------|
| *Reading* | | | |
| Real word reading | 82.8 | 90.6 | 89.8 |
| % Correct | (12.7) | (6.3) | (7.5) |
| Nonword reading | 44.9 | 60.5 | 85.8 |
| % Correct | (16.2) | (15.3) | (12.5) |
| *Spelling* | | | |
| Real word spelling | 65.7 | 73.1 | 66.3 |
| % Correct | (14.7) | (8.7) | (13.7) |
| Nonword spelling | 27.9 | 40.4 | 47.3 |
| % Correct | (13.9) | (14.9) | (16.4) |

## Discussion

The performance of the Hong Kong University students without training in phonetics on the phonological awareness tasks is very like that of people diagnosed as having specific reading disability. Nevertheless, their ability to read and spell real words was not impaired compared with the other two groups of students who had learned written English as a second language. Group 1 subjects' results were similar to those reported for the phonologically dyslexic case of RE (Campbell and Butterworth, 1985). RE was also highly literate but had unusual difficulty with nonwords. In contrast, nonwords presented no difficulty for the Guangzhou students whose learning of an alphabetic script when acquiring written Chinese had allowed the development of phonological awareness skills. Group 2, Hong Kong students who had completed two years of phonetic training at the tertiary level, provided an interesting control. Their results suggest that although it is possible subsequently to acquire some phonological awareness skills, the influence of learning their first written language logographically was still apparent in their poor performance on phoneme segmentation and visual rhyme identification.

The frequently quoted statement that we 'only learn to read once' (Saville-Troike, 1976: 87) highlights the expectation that skills learned in one language will be transferred to another. Different orthographies represent their units of phonology differently. For example, Chinese characters represent one-syllable morphemes, not phonemes. Since phonological awareness develops in relation to orthography (Huang and Hanley, 1994; Read et al., 1986), literacy in different orthographies results in differences in phonological awareness. Chinese students who learn an alphabetic script (pinyin) when acquiring written Chinese (Group 3) are able to assemble phonology from letters and have a superior knowledge of the sound structure of the language and the skill to manipulate sounds. The phonological awareness derived from Chinese orthography learned as logographs affects the acquisition of English as a written language in that students' poor phonological awareness skills limited their ability to read and spell unknown words. Their reading strategy in English leads to performance on tests of phonological awareness and nonword reading and spelling that resembles the symptoms associated with specific reading disability or phonological dyslexia.

It is not appropriate, however, to classify the Group 1 subjects as phonologically dyslexic, because there is no underlying developmental or acquired deficit. RE , for example, was not able to develop phonological awareness even when she was given explicit analytic reading instruction as a child, so she was taught by the 'look and say' method because of her disorder. In contrast, the Group 1 subjects probably would have acquired phonological awareness if they had been taught an alphabetic system in an analytic way (similar to students in Group 3). Their phonological awareness deficit, that mimics disorder, only exists because they had not been exposed to phonemic segmentation.

Another example of symptomatology in the absence of impairment is provided by the next experiment.

## Experiment two

When children start to speak they make errors of pronunciation. Particular error patterns have been identified as being typical of normal development (Smith, 1973; Grunwell, 1982). Other error patterns are associated with disordered phonological acquisition (Dunn and Davis, 1983). Children making these error patterns fail to acquire speech normally at the appropriate age and are at risk for later literacy learning difficulties (Dodd et al., 1994). While many normal developmental error patterns are common across languages (Bortolini and Leonard, 1991) some are specific to particular languages. Young English and Cantonese children both substitute continuants with plosives (e.g. [tɪp] *ship*) and 'front' velar consonants (e.g. [tʌp] *cup*). However, Cantonese-speaking children make some errors that are atypical of phonological acquisition in English. For example, So and Dodd (in press) found that the way in which Cantonese-speaking children realise clusters shows two subtle patterns not commonly found in children acquiring English:

1.  Younger children's most common realisation of /k$^{(h)}$w/ was [k$^{(h)}$]. If the /k/ was fronted it was more likely to be realised as a [p] than as a [t] (e.g. [pa] /kwa/), whereas a singleton /k/ was usually fronted to [t], and never to [p] (e.g. [tɐj] /kɐj/). Thus, although the /w/ was deleted, many children took account of its place of articulation in choosing how to mark the cluster. A similar error pattern is

**not** reported for English-speaking children: place of articulation of the deleted member does not influence choice of substitute (e.g. [pin] *queen* would be an unusual error).

2. When older children reduce clusters they often mark the level of aspiration of the target cluster by realising /kw/ as [f] but /k⁽ʰ⁾w/ as [p⁽ʰ⁾]. Although English does not have contrastive aspiration, it does have a voicing distinction which is analogous in that both aspiration and voicing are measurable in terms of voice onset time (VOT). Level of voicing does not appear to influence the cluster reduction pattern of English-speaking children, e.g. *trip* and *drip* → [tɪp] and [dɪp].

One question arising from the differing normal developmental error patterns in English and Cantonese concerns how children acquiring both English and Cantonese reconcile the two phonological systems. Do they have one phonological output system that serves both languages, producing the same error patterns in both languages? Or, do the speech errors they make in each language reflect error patterns typical of mono-lingual children?

## Method

### Subjects

Sixteen children who attended a weekly Sunday afternoon school (The Chinese School, Newcastle upon Tyne, UK) participated in the study. All were born in Britain to Cantonese-speaking immigrants and Cantonese was their dominant language. Most attended preschools where English was spoken. Cantonese was the primary language spoken at home for all children, but they were also exposed to English since one or both parents and elder siblings sometimes addressed the children in English. The children were also exposed to English through television. The children were aged between 25 and 51 months. There were nine girls and seven boys in the group. Their parents had a range of occupations (e.g. catering, university lecturing, and dentistry).

### Materials

The children were asked to name pictures in both Cantonese and English. The Cantonese Segmental Phonology Test (So, 1992), which consists of 31 pictures whose names elicit all consonant and vowel phonemes of Cantonese at least once, was administered. This test has been normed on a large sample of monolingual Cantonese-speaking children in Hong Kong (So and Dodd, in press). Additional pictures were used to elicit productions in English of /kw/ clusters in the words *queen*, *quiet, quick* and *squirrel*. Children were also asked to name, in English, other pictures to clarify their phonological error patterns for English sounds not sampled by the pictures in the Cantonese Segmental Phonology Test.

## Procedure

The children were tested individually by a Cantonese–English bilingual teacher who was familiar to all the children. They were asked to name the pictures first in Cantonese, and then in English. The children's productions were audiotaped and later transcribed by one Cantonese speaker and a phonetician specialising in the phonetic transcription of speech disorder. Only spontaneous namings were included in the analyses of the data, except for imitations of some of the English words containing /kw/ clusters, and the productions of the youngest child who was often unwilling to name spontaneously the pictures in English.

## Results

### Quantitative analyses

Paired *t*-testing revealed that:

- The children pronounced fewer of the words correctly when naming them in Cantonese than in English ($t(15) = 3.52$, $p < 0.01$).
- The percentage of phonemes produced correctly in the Cantonese trial was less than that for the English trial ($t(15) = 3.51$, $p < 0.01$).
- Despite fewer English words being produced, the number of phonemes included in the Cantonese sample (mean 88.9) did not differ from that of the English sample (mean 98.1).
- The children's phoneme repertoires, based on at least one correct production, were age-appropriate compared with monolingual norms, except for the youngest child who was missing one Cantonese phoneme she should have acquired.

### Qualitative analysis: error patterns

Table 6.3 shows that a high proportion of errors affected vowel phonemes. This is surprising since monolingual children rarely make vowel errors after two years of age. Table 6.4 provides a list of the phonological error patterns in Cantonese and English under three headings:

**Table 6.3** Quantitative summary of Cantonese and English error data

|           | % Words in error | % Phoneme errors | % of Errors: vowels | No response | Number of Phones missing |
|-----------|------------------|------------------|---------------------|-------------|--------------------------|
| Cantonese | 24.33            | 9.87             | 8.14                | 0.25        | 0.81                     |
|           | 6.5 – 65.5       | 2.2–29.9         | 0 – 34.8            | 0 – 2       | 0 – 6                    |
| English   | 13.16            | 5.23             | 26.15               | 7.5         | 0.5                      |
|           | 0 –71.4          | 0 – 26.7         | 0 –100              | 0 –18       | 0 – 4                    |

*Expected*: those typical and age-appropriate according to norms for monolingual children;
*Delayed*: those typical of monolingual development but inappropriate for chronological age;
*Atypical*: error patterns associated with disorder in monolingual children.

**Table 6.4** Expected, delayed and atypical error patterns in Cantonese and English (number of children evidencing the error pattern)

| Cantonese | English |
|-----------|---------|
| *Expected* | |
| Final consonant deletion (2) | Final consonant deletion (1) |
| Stopping (3) | Stopping (1) |
| Fronting (4) | Fronting (1) |
| Affrication/Frication (1) | Cluster reduction (2) |
| Deaspiration (1) | Weak syllable deletion (2) |
| Deaffrication (1) | Gliding (3) |
|  | Voicing (1) |
|  | Consonant harmony (2) |
| *Delayed* | |
| Final consonant deletion (9) | Final consonant deletion (7) |
| Fronting (4) | Fronting (3) |
| Affrication/Frication (4) | Cluster reduction (10) |
| Deaffrication (5) | Consonant harmony (1) |
| Consonant harmony (3) | Weak syllable deletion (1) |
|  | Voicing (2) |
| *Atypical* | |
| Initial consonant deletion (3) | Initial consonant deletion (1) |
| Voicing (8) | Backing (2) |
| Backing (7) | Deaffrication (2) |
| Aspiration (4) | Affrication (2) |
| Addition (7) | Addition (2) |
| Gliding (4) | Nasalisation (1) |
|  | Transposition (1) |

*Comparison with monolingual Cantonese-speaking children*

A number of the bilingual children's error patterns showed delayed suppression of normal developmental error patterns, for example:

- deaffrication [tiu] /tsiu/ *banana*;
- fronting [tʰɐm] /kʰɐm/ *piano*;
- affrication [tsɐi min] /sɐi min/ *washing face*;
- consonant harmony [nin wa] /tin wa/] *telephone*.

Overall, three-quarters of the children showed delayed development of some aspects of their Cantonese phonological system. Only one child failed to use any atypical phonological error patterns. Less than 10% of the monolingual sample (So and Dodd, in press) used the error patterns listed in the *Atypical* section of Table 6.4 (such as initial consonant deletion, e.g. [in wa] /tin wa/ *telephone;* backing, e.g. [kʰɐn] /kʰɐm/ *piano*). Two other error patterns, observed in 44% of the bilingual sample, were voicing (e.g. [dzuk] /tsuk/ *porridge*) and addition of sounds (e.g. [toun] /tou/ *knife*). Neither of these patterns were observed in any of the 268 children in the monolingual sample.

*Comparison with monolingual English speaking children*

Three quarters of the bilingual children used some error patterns typical of monolingual phonological acquisition in English that were inappropriate for chronological age, for example:

- final consonant deletion [bɪskə] *biscuit*;
- fronting [tændəl] *candle*;
- weak syllable deletion [nanəz] *bananas*;
- consonant harmony [ʃɪʃ] *fish*.

A typical phonological error patterns were exhibited by 38% of the children:

- affrication [tsʌŋ] *tongue*;
- addition [ŋai] *eye*;
- backing [sɔk] *skirt*;
- deaffrication [pɒrɪʃ] *porridge*;
- nasalisation [æpən] *apple*.

*Comparison of Cantonese and English phonological rules*

Inspection of Table 6.4 suggests that despite Cantonese being the first language of the children, it is more susceptible to delayed and atypical phonological error patterns than is their English phonological system. A Friedman non-parametric Analysis of Variance was used to compare the number of delayed error patterns exhibited by the children in Cantonese and English. It was not significant ($F(1) = 0.63, p = 0.803$). However, a similar analysis of the number of atypical error patterns used by the children in Cantonese and English was significant ($F(1) = 9.0, p < 0.01$). These results indicated that the children were significantly more likely to exhibit atypical error patterns in Cantonese than in English. However, relatively few of the error patterns were used in both languages. The mean number of error patterns per child common to both English and Cantonese was 0.88, whereas the mean number of error patterns apparent in only one language was 4.2.

## Discussion

The results indicated that the children's phonological error patterns were different for their two emerging languages. These error patterns also reflected delay or were atypical of monolingual children's developmental errors. Delayed phonological acquisition is probably not surprising given the need to master two phonological systems in the preschool years and, perhaps proportionately less exposure to each language compared with monolingual children. Further, other studies have also reported delayed development of receptive vocabulary and specific aspects of syntax in French–English bilingual children (e.g. Doyle, Champagne and Segalowitz, 1978). However, the observation of so many atypical error patterns was unexpected. Many of these error patterns (e.g. initial consonant deletion, backing, aspiration, frication) are associated with phonological disorder in English (Dodd, 1995) and Cantonese (So and Dodd, 1994). A longitudinal study would be needed to establish that the 15 children in the sample who evidenced atypical error patterns were not phonologically disordered. However, it seems unlikely that this would be so, given an incidence rate for phonological disorder of about 5% for English speaking children (Enderby and Philipp, 1986). Rather, it seems plausible that a bilingual language learning environment results in the development of unusual speech error patterns which should not be considered to be the result of an impairment, despite reflecting the symptoms of phonological disorder.

Most studies of bilingual children have focused on syntax and semantics, rather than phonology (Watson, 1991). Nevertheless phonological 'mixing' (combining elements of both phonologies) has been reported in case studies of young bilingual children which gives rise to atypical speech errors (Burling, 1959; Fantini, 1979; Mulford and Hecht, 1979; de Houwer, 1995). Watson's (1991: 44) review of phonological data from the few available case studies led him to conclude that, 'Differentiation, avoidance of interference, learning to categorise acoustic input in two contrasting ways are all tasks which must be carried out by the bilingual and which the monolingual escapes. Obviously, all of these assume a degree of mental processing, involving strategies which will remain undeveloped in those exposed to only one language.' However, given that the number of children and languages investigated is few and that the analyses often focused on order of phoneme acquisition rather than error patterns, previous research provides no explanation for the present results. By default, then, we can only say our data support Duncan's (1989: 3) claim that, 'The bilingual speaker is not a monolingual speaker times two.'

## Conclusions

The results from the two experiments presented indicate that bilingual individuals, with no history of an impairment, behave similarly to monolingual people who have been diagnosed as phonologically disordered. The findings have implications for theory of bilingual language acquisition and understanding the nature of the deficits underlying monolingual children's phonological disorder.

Children who have a specific reading disability associated with a phonological deficit are unable to derive the rules governing the relationship between spoken and written productions of words because their ability to parse the phonological system of their language is disordered. The nature of the impairment is probably different for different children. Some might have deficits in auditory processing (Tallal, Miller and Fitch, 1993), others in the ability to abstract rules per se (Gillon, 1995), or representation and processing of information in short-term memory (Gathercole and Baddeley, 1990). Nevertheless, the deficit limits the information available to the mental system used for performing tasks assessing phonological awareness. In contrast, children who have learned their first written language as logographs do not need to establish the phonological assembly route, and the phonological awareness skills required to parse an alphabetic script are therefore unavailable. However, explicit training in parsing, provided by training in phonetics, allows at least the partial development of phonological assembly skills in people who have learned their first written language as logographs, indicating that it is experience that determines performance. Perhaps one clinical implication of this argument is that some children currently diagnosed as having specific reading disability because of their poor phonological awareness skills might be suffering from lack of appropriate experience rather than an impairment.

The acquisition of phonological error patterns by bilingual children which are not typical of those made by monolingual children may also be accounted for in terms of the nature of the information available to the mental mechanism that processes phonological signals. Irrespective of whether developmental phonological errors are explained in terms of connectionist (Jusczyk, 1992) or generative (Smith, 1973) theory, theorists agree that there is a cognitive mechanism that allows children to parse heard speech and derive an understanding of the constraints that limit how speech sounds may be combined to make up words in a particular language. When children are exposed to two languages where those constraints differ markedly, as is the case with Cantonese and English phonologies, it could be predicted that atypical error patterns might arise. For example, the predominant word form in Cantonese is the open syllable (CV) whereas many English syllables are closed (CVC). It is hardly surprising then that some of the bilingual children consistently added a syllable final consonant to Cantonese words, nor that the consonant chosen came from the repertoire of speech sounds allowable in syllable final position in Cantonese phonology. The characteristics of the developmental errors of bilingual children are similar to those of children who seem to have an impaired cognitive–linguistic ability to analyse input (Dodd and McCormack, 1995). Thus, irrespective of the reason why input to the cognitive mechanism governing spoken output differs from that of normal monolingual children, similar error patterns arise.

How does this interpretation of the findings bear on the assumption that it is possible to better understand the nature of normal language function by describing the effects of specific types of impairment? The symptoms described as being associated with impairment (poor performance on phonological awareness tasks, atypical speech error patterns) can also be observed in unimpaired people who have bilingual language learning experience. That is, the symptoms do not *only* arise as a direct result of an impairment. Rather, it might be argued that atypical performance might result from the nature of the information which is available to be processed by a normally functioning cognitive mechanism. In the case of bilingual people, exposure to two differing orthographies and/or phonological systems (anomalous input) might influence their understanding of the rules that govern those language modes. In contrast, phonologically disordered monolingual people's understanding of the rules that govern spoken and written language would be constrained by their deficit in parsing phonological information (anomalous processing). The finding that similar performance arises in both cases suggests that the relationship between impairment and the symptoms of disorder may be more complex than has previously been acknowledged.

## Acknowledgements

We are grateful to the children and parents for their cooperation; to the students and their clinical supervisors; and to the CRCG, University of

Hong Kong, the University of Newcastle and the Australian NH&MRC for financial assistance. Ruth Campbell and Alison Holm commented on earlier drafts.

# References

Barnitz, J.G. (1978). *Interrelationship of Orthography and Phonological Structure in Learning to Read* (Technical Report No 57). Champaign: University of Illinois, Centre for the Study of Reading. (ERIC Document Reproduction Service No ED 150 546).

Bortolini, U. and Leonard, L. (1991). The speech of phonologically disordered children acquiring Italian. *Clinical Linguistics and Phonetics*, **5**, 1–12.

Burling, R. (1959/1971). Language development of a Garo and English speaking child. *Word*, **15**, 45–68. Reprinted in A. Bar-Ado and W. Leopold (Eds) *Child Language*, pp. 170–185. Englewood Cliffs, NJ: Prentice-Hall.

Campbell, R. and Butterworth, B. (1985). Phonological dyslexia and dysgraphia in a highly literate subject: a developmental case with associated deficits of phonemic processing and awareness. *Quarterly Journal of Experimental Psychology*, **37A**, 435–475.

de Houwer, A. (1995). *The Acquisition of Two Languages from Birth: A Case Study*. Cambridge: The University Press.

Dodd, B. (1995). *Differential Diagnosis and Treatment of Children with Speech Disorder*. London: Whurr.

Dodd, B. and McCormack, P. (1995). Differential diagnosis of phonological disorders. In B. Dodd (Ed.) *Differential Diagnosis and Treatment of Children with Speech Disorder*, pp. 65–90. London: Whurr.

Dodd, B., Gillon, G., Oerlemans, M., Russell, T., Syrmis, M. and Wilson, H. (1995). Phonological disorder and the acquisition of literacy. In B. Dodd (Ed.) *Differential Diagnosis and Treatment of Children with Speech Disorder*, pp. 125–147. London: Whurr.

Dodd, B., Leahy, J. and Hambly, G. (1989). Phonological disorders in children: underlying cognitive deficits. *British Journal of Developmental Psychology*, **7**, 55–71.

Doyle, A.-B., Champagne, M. and Segalowitz, N. (1978). Some issues in the assessment of linguistic consequences of early bilingualism. In M. Paradis (Ed.) *Aspects of Bilingualism*, pp. 13–20. Columbia: Hornbeam Press.

Duncan, D. (1989). *Working with Bilingual Language Disability*. London: Chapman & Hall.

Dunn, C. and Davis, B. (1983). Phonological process occurrence in phonologically disordered children. *Applied Psycholinguistics*, **4**, 187–207.

Enderby, P. and Philipp, R. (1986). Speech and language handicap: towards knowing the size of the problem. *British Journal of Disorders of Communication*, **21**, 151–165.

Fantini, A. (1979). *Language Acquisition of a Bilingual Child*. Clevedon: Multilingual Matters.

Gathercole, S. and Baddeley, A. (1990). Phonological memory deficits in language disordered children: Is there a causal connection? *Journal of Memory and Language*, **29**, 336–360.

Gillon, G. (1995). *The Phonological, Semantic and Syntactic Skills of Children with Specific Reading Disability*. Unpublished PhD Thesis, The University of Queensland.

Gillon, G. and Dodd, B. (1994). A prospective study of the relationship between phonological, semantic and syntactic skills and specific reading disability. *Reading and Writing*, 6, 321–345.

Grunwell, P. (1982). *Clinical Phonology*. London: Croom Helm.

Huang, H. and Hanley, J.R. (1994). Phonological awareness and visual skills in learning to read Chinese and English. *Cognition*, 54, 73–98.

Jusczyk, P. (1992). Developing phonological categories from the speech signal. In C. Ferguson, L. Menn and C. Stoel-Gammon (Eds) *Phonological Development: Models, Research, Implications*, pp. 17–64. Timonium: York Press.

Leitao, S., Hogben, J. and Fletcher, J. (1995). Predicting literacy difficulties: investigating the relationship between phonological performance and phonological processing. *Australian Association of Speech and Hearing Conference*, Brisbane.

Leong, C.K. (1973). Hong Kong. In J. Downing (Ed.) *Comparative Reading: Cross-National Studies of Behaviour and Processes in Reading and Writing*, pp. 383–402. New York: Macmillan.

Mulford, R. and Hecht, B. (1979). Learning to speak without an accent: acquisition of a second language. *4th Annual Conference on Language Development*, Boston University.

Perin, D. (1983). Phonemic segmentation and spelling. *British Journal of Psychology*, 74, 9–44.

Rack, J., Snowling, M. and Olsen, R. (1992). The nonword reading deficit in developmental dyslexia: a review. *Reading Research Quarterly*, 27, 29–53.

Read, C., Zhang, Y., Nie, H. and Ding, B. (1986). The ability to manipulate speech sounds depends on knowing alphabetic spelling. *Cognition*, 24, 31–44.

Saville-Troike, M. (1976). *Foundations for Teaching English as a Second Language: Theory and Method for Multicultural Education*. Englewood Cliffs, NJ: Prentice-Hall.

Smith, N. (1973). *The Acquisition of Phonology: A Case Study*. Cambridge: The University Press.

So, L.K.H. (1992). *Cantonese Segmental Phonology Test (Research Version)*. Hong Kong: The University Department of Speech and Hearing Sciences.

So, L.K.H. and Dodd, B. (1994). Phonologically disordered Cantonese-speaking children. *Clinical Linguistics and Phonetics*, 8, 235–255.

So, L.K.H. and Dodd, B. (in press). Cantonese-speaking children's acquisition of phonology. *Journal of Child Language*.

Taft, M. and Chen, H.-C. (1992). Judging homophony in Chinese: the influence of tones. In H.C. Chen and O.J. Tzeng (Eds) *Language Processing in Chinese*, pp. 151–172. Amsterdam: Elsevier Science.

Tallal, P., Miller, S. and Fitch, R.H. (1993). Neurobiological basis of speech: a case for the preeminence of temporal processing. In P. Tallal, A. Galaburda, R. Llinas and C. von Euler (Eds) *Temporal Information Processing in the Nervous System*, pp. 27–47. New York: Academy of Sciences.

Watson, I. (1991). Phonological processing in two languages. In E. Bialystok (Ed.) *Language Processing in Bilingual Children*, pp. 25–48. Cambridge: The University Press.

World Health Organization (1980) .*International Classification of Impairment, Disability and Handicap*. Geneva: WHO.

# Chapter 7
# The Role of Subcortical Structures in Language: Clinico-neuroradiological Studies of Brain-damaged Subjects

BRUCE E MURDOCH

## Abstract

*Contemporary models of the role of subcortical structures in language are largely based on the findings of clinico-anatomical studies that have investigated the language abilities of subjects with subcortical lesion sites. The aim of this chapter is to review and evaluate the current theories of subcortical participation in language generated by investigations of brain–behaviour relationships along classical clinico-anatomical lines. In recent years, the development of these subcortical models has been extensively influenced by the development and intro-duction of new neuro-imaging techniques. Consequently, as part of the process of evaluating these models, the evidence gained from clinico-neuroradiological correlation studies supporting a role for structures such as the thalamus and corpus striatum in language will be presented and discussed. Further, contemporary models will be evalu-ated with reference to the predicted and reported language abilities of subjects with lesions of the thalamus or striatum or their subcortical connections to the cortical language areas*

## Introduction

The cerebral cortex has traditionally been considered the neural substrate of language. According to the classical 'associationist' anatomo-functional models of language function proposed by Wernicke (1874) and Lichtheim (1885), subcortical lesions could only produce language deficits if they disrupted the association pathways that connect the various cortical language centres. Over the past two decades, however, this traditional view of the cerebral cortex as the neural substrate of language has been challenged by the findings of a proliferating number of clinico-neuroradiological correlation studies. In particular, the introduction during this period of new neuroradiological methods for lesion localisation *in vivo*, including computed tomography (CT) and more recently, magnetic resonance imaging (MRI), has led to an increasing number of reports in the literature of aphasia following apparently purely subcortical lesions. Lesions involving the striato-capsular region (Damasio, Damasio, Rizzo, Varney and Gersh, 1982; Kennedy and Murdoch, 1989; Murdoch, Kennedy, McCallum and Siddle, 1991; Naeser, Alexander, Helm-Estabrooks, Levine, Laughlin and Geschwind, 1982; Wallesch, 1985), the thalamus (Bogousslavsky, Regli and Uske, 1988; Graff-Radford, Eslinger, Damasio and Yamada, 1984; McFarling, Rothi and Heilman, 1982; Murdoch, 1987) or the periventricular white matter (PVWM) (Alexander, Naeser and Palumbo, 1987; Naeser et al., 1982; Naeser, Palumbo, Helm-Estabrooks, Stiassny-Eder and Albert, 1989) have all been reported to produce aphasia. Consequently, in recent years there has been growing acceptance of a role for subcortical structures in language.

One outcome of the reported clinico-neuroradiological correlation studies has been the development of a number of theories regarding the function of subcortical structures in language. These theories, largely developed on the basis of speech and language data collected from subjects who have had cerebrovascular accidents involving the thalamus or striato-capsular region, have been expressed as neuroanatomically-based language processing models (Alexander et al., 1987; Crosson, 1985; Wallesch and Papagno, 1988). The aim of the present chapter is to evaluate these contemporary models of subcortical participation in language with reference to the predicted and reported language abilities of subjects with lesions of the thalamus or striato-capsular region. Prior to examining these models, however, it is necessary to revise briefly the neuroanatomy of the subcortical structures and to review the nature of the language deficits reported to occur in association with either thalamic or striato-capsular lesions.

## Neuroanatomy of the striato-capsular region and thalamus

Rather than being localised in definite cortical areas, contemporary theories propose that language is subserved by a complex circuit which links cortical and subcortical structures (Alexander and Crutcher, 1990; Alexander, DeLong and Strick, 1986). In particular, some authors have proposed that cortico-striato-pallido-thalamo-cortical loops are involved in language (Crosson, 1985; Wallesch and Papagno, 1988). Consequently, prior to examining recent models of subcortical participation in language, it is important that the reader be provided with a basic understanding of the neuroanatomy of the principal subcortical structures and their connections.

**Neuroanatomy of the striato-capsular region**

The striato-capsular region occupies the deep, central portion of each cerebral hemisphere and comprises the basal ganglia and internal capsule. Anatomically, the basal ganglia consist of the caudate nucleus, the putamen, the globus pallidus and the amygdaloid nucleus. Some neuroanatomists also include the claustrum as part of the basal ganglia. Collectively, the globus pallidus and the putamen are referred to as the lenticular nucleus (lentiform nucleus). The lenticular nucleus combined with the caudate nucleus make up what is known as the corpus striatum (from here on referred to as the striatum), so called because of the striated (striped) nature of this region.

Complex connections exist between the various individual nuclei of the basal ganglia and between the nuclei and other brain structures, including the cerebral cortex and thalamus. Briefly, the afferent inflow to the striatum is mainly from the massive cortico-striatal pathways which project fibres to the caudate nucleus and putamen from nearly all parts of the cerebral cortex, but especially from the motor areas. The precentral motor cortex is mainly connected with the putamen (Tanridag and Kirshner, 1987) and, the associative areas of the prefrontal, temporal and parietal cortex are primarily linked with the caudate nucleus (Goldman-Rakic, 1984). Both Broca's and Wernicke's language areas allegedly project onto the same area in the head of the caudate nucleus (Damasio et al., 1982). The striatum also receives projections from the substantia nigra (nigro-striatal pathways) and primary non-specific nuclei of the thalamus (Alexander and Crutcher, 1990; Tanridag and Kirshner, 1987). From the caudate nucleus and putamen, the input is relayed to the globus pallidus. The globus pallidus then sends projections to the substantia nigra (pallido-nigral pathways), the subthalamic nucleus (pallido-subthalamic pathways), and to the ventral anterior, ventral lateral and non-specific nuclei of the thalamus (pallido-thalamic pathways). Since the ventral anterior nucleus of the thalamus projects its output to the motor and pre-motor cortex, an important circuit is established between the motor cortex, striatum, thalamus and motor cortex again, i.e. the cortico-striato-pallido-thalamo-cortical loop. It is important to note that there are no major white matter pathways connecting the striatum directly back to the cerebral cortex. Consequently, any influence that the striatum has on cortical function must occur via the thalamus using the above loop (Wallesch and Papagno, 1988). Alexander et al. (1986) noted the presence of at least five cortico-striato-pallido-thalamo-cortical loops which participate in motor, cognitive and other associated functions. These loops, although structurally and functionally different circuits, are essentially parallel in structure and connect the basal ganglia and thalamus to separate regions of the cortex (Alexander and Crutcher, 1990; Alexander et al. 1986). Within each loop, the striatum receives multiple cortico-striatal inputs only from cortical areas that are functionally related, and in most cases, interconnected. Although the role of these loops remains speculative, loops of this kind have been regarded by some authors as being important in language (Brunner, Kornhuber, Seemuller, Suger and Wallesch, 1982; Crosson, 1985; Wallesch and Papagno, 1988). The possible role of these loops in language is discussed further below.

### Neuroanatomy of the thalamus

The thalamus is a large mass of grey matter located above the midbrain and medial to the posterior limb of the internal capsule. It forms part of the diencephalon and consists of more than 30 anatomically and functionally different nuclei. The internal medullary lamina divides the thalamus into groups of nuclei including the anterior nuclei, ventral anterior nuclei, ventral lateral nuclei, ventral postero-lateral nuclei, pulvinar, medial nuclei (Tanridag and Krishner, 1987) and non-specific intralaminar and midline nuclei (Wallesch and Papagno, 1988).

The thalamus has multiple connections with both higher and lower structures in the central nervous system. The ventral lateral nucleus and the ventral anterior nucleus are specific motor nuclei in the sense that they receive information from the cerebellum, corpus striatum and substantia nigra and project to motor areas in the frontal lobe. The ventral lateral nuclei mainly project to the motor cortex and the ventral anterior nuclei to the premotor cortex (Tanridag and Kirshner, 1987). The ventral posterior nucleus is a specific sensory nucleus and functions as a thalamic relay for general sensation. It receives input from ascending sensory systems and projects fibres to the secondary somesthetic cortex located on the post central gyrus via the posterior limb of the internal capsule.

Bidirectional fibres connect the pulvinar nuclei of the thalamus with the temporoparietal association cortex including Wernicke's area (Wallesch and Papagno, 1988). Non-specific thalamic nuclei allow communication between the reticular formation of the brainstem and the cortex and act to transmit cortically arousing information. The reticular formation receives information directly and indirectly from spinoreticular tracts, spino-thalamic tracts, spino-tectal tracts, auditory tracts and visual tracts so that almost any sensory stimulus in the body can activate it. The non-specific thalamo-cortical system is regarded as the uppermost end of the reticular formation which acts to control the level of activation of the cerebral cortex (Guyton, 1981).

# Language disorders associated with subcortical lesions

The clinical picture with regard to the nature of the language impairment varies greatly in subcortical aphasia. One general comment that applies to the majority of the language disturbances associated with subcortical lesions is that they are often 'atypical', not fitting neatly into any of the classic aphasia syndromes defined by classical Bostonian taxonomy. Most authors agree, however, that aphasia associated with thalamic lesions has features which distinguish it from aphasia occurring in association with striato-capsular lesions. The evidence available suggests that lesions involving the thalamus produce language deficits through different pathophysiological mechanisms than other subcortical lesions (Graff-Radford et al., 1984). Certainly, given that the thalamus and striato-capsular region have differing blood supplies, they can each be independently affected by cerebrovascular accidents.

### Aphasia associated with striato-capsular lesions

Striato-capsular lesions of the dominant hemisphere can be associated with varying degrees of language impairment, ranging from relatively normal language abilities through to severe impairment in language tasks such as spontaneous speech, naming, repetition, auditory and reading comprehension and writing (Alexander and LoVerme, 1980; Damasio et al., 1982; Vallar, Papagno and Cappa, 1988; Yang, Yang, Pan, Lai and Yang, 1989). Although not uniform in their language presentation, depending upon their site of lesion, three different patterns of language impairment have been reported to occur in the acute stage following striato-capsular lesions. Anterior lesions of the basal ganglia and internal capsule may result in a Broca's-type, a transcortical motor-type aphasia or a dysarthric/aphemic disorder (Damasio et al., 1982; Naeser et al., 1982). Posterior striato-capsular lesions have been reported to cause a Wernicke's-type of aphasia, whereas lesions involving both the anterior and posterior regions of the basal ganglia/internal capsule may lead to global aphasia (Alexander et al., 1987; Naeser et al., 1982). Exceptions to these patterns, however, do exist (Robin and Schienberg, 1990).

### Aphasia associated with thalamic lesions

Aphasia associated with thalamic lesions appears to be much more homogeneous than the language impairment associated with striato-capsular lesions. Although some variability in the language profile does exist, a number of authors believe that thalamic aphasia has enough defining characteristics to warrant its identification as a 'new' aphasic syndrome. Despite this, thalamic aphasia does not fall into any of the currently accepted cortical aphasias. Overall, the language disturbance appears to resemble a transcortical aphasia (Alexander and LoVerme, 1980; Cappa and Vignolo, 1979; Chesson, 1983; McFarling et al., 1982).

The features of thalamic aphasia most commonly reported include: preserved repetition; variable but often relatively good auditory comprehension; a reduction in spontaneous speech; naming impairments with paraphasias (semantic and phonemic), neologisms, circumlocutions and jargon being produced; perseveration; impaired writing abilities; and fading or lowered voice volume (Aten, White and Pribram, 1982; Bougousslavsky et al., 1988; Bruyn, 1989; Robin and Schienberg, 1984; and Yang et al., 1989).

# Role of subcortical structures in language

Although there is growing acceptance that brain lesions involving the subcortical structures of the dominant hemisphere can cause aphasia, the role of subcortical structures in language remains speculative and poorly understood. Evidence to support a role for structures such as the striatum and thalamus in language comes from three main sources: firstly, from clinico-anatomical observations of language disordered subjects with subcortical lesions primarily of vascular origin (Alexander et al., 1987; Brunner et al., 1982; Cappa et al., 1983; Kennedy and Murdoch, 1993; Valler et al., 1988); secondly, in the case of the thalamus, from studies involving electrical stimulation of the thalamus during surgical operations (Fedio and Van Buren, 1975; Ojemann, 1977) or surgically induced thalamic lesions (Riklan and Levita, 1970); thirdly, from anatomical studies that have demonstrated extensive white matter pathways linking the subcortical structures and the language areas of the cerebral cortex.

On the basis of the evidence gained from these sources, several theories have been proposed to explain the role of subcortical structures in language. Among the first to attribute a language role to the dominant thalamus were Penfield and Roberts (1959). They suggested that the thalamus, specifically the pulvinar, is responsible for mediation between the anterior (Broca's area) and posterior (Wernicke's area) language centres, thereby playing a role in the integration of language. Their suggestion was based on the presence of strong fibre connections between the pulvinar and the temporo-parietal cortex and the parallel evolutionary expansion of the pulvinar and speech cortex over the mammalian species.

Ojemann and colleagues (Mateer and Ojemann, 1983; Ojemann, 1975, 1976; Ojemann and Ward, 1971) have suggested that the thalamus acts as an 'altering system' for the cortical language areas and that aphasia associated with thalamic lesions is the outcome of deficient arousal of otherwise intact cortical language mechanisms. These proposals were based on the results of experiments involving stimulation of the thalamus prior to stereotaxic lesions of that structure. Specifically, Ojemann and Ward (1971) and Ojemann (1976) suggested that the dominant lateral thalamus may be involved in producing a 'specific alerting response' which directs attention to the external environment while simultaneously inhibiting retrieval of already internalised material. Similarly, Fedio and Van Buren (1975) proposed that not all incoming sensory information (visual or from short-term memory) is allowed access to cortical regions. Thus the thalamus may act to alert the cortex to important incoming information while blocking/gating other less important input.

Rather than a specific linguistic activating effect as proposed by Ojemann and colleagues, Mohr, Watters and Duncan (1975) suggested that the thalamus may be involved in non-specific regulation of cortical activity. Both Mohr et al. (1975) and Luria (1977) believed that the language system of thalamic aphasics was unimpaired, and that non-linguistic factors (e.g. reduced cortical tone, impaired gating/blocking processes) resulted in the language deficits associated with thalamic lesions. Indeed, Luria (1977) suggested that the language disorder observed in his thalamic patients was in fact a 'quasi-aphasia'.

Based on the observed predominance of semantic paraphasias in cases of thalamic aphasia, some authors have suggested a semantic role for the thalamus in language (Alexander and LoVerme, 1980; Cappa and Vignolo, 1979). Crosson (1985) suggested that the thalamus provides a mechanism through which the temporo-parietal area of the cerebral cortex, involved in semantic and phonological decoding, monitors the encoding of language in the anterior language area prior to execution of encoded material in speech. In particular, Crosson (1985) proposed that reciprocal connections between the anterior cortical and temporo-parietal areas which pass through the thalamus provide the means by which the temporo-parietal cortex checks the language encoded in the anterior cortex for semantic accuracy. Crosson's model of subcortical participation in language is explained in more detail below.

The role played by the basal ganglia in language is even more speculative than that of the thalamus. Nonetheless, the data that are available do allow for the formulation of tentative hypotheses regarding the role of the striatum in language. Not least among these data is the anatomical position of the basal ganglia relative to the cortex and thalamus. As outlined previously, the putamen and caudate nucleus receive input primarily from the cortex, but these structures do not send any output directly to the cortex. Most output from the striatum is mediated through the globus pallidus which sends numerous fibre connections to the ventral anterior and ventral lateral nuclei of the thalamus.

The basal ganglia have been considered to be involved in non-linguistic and linguistic programme generation including activation of the cortex (Crosson, 1985; Luria, 1977; Mesulam, 1981; Robin and Schienberg, 1990), sequencing of cortical information (Metter et al., 1988) and integration of cortical information (Damasio et al., 1982; Penfield and Roberts, 1959; Riklan and Cooper, 1975; Robin and Schienberg, 1990; Wallesch and Papagno, 1988). A specific motor release mechanism for speech, controlled by the basal ganglia, has also been proposed (Crosson, 1985).

Further consideration of the specific roles of subcortical structures in language are provided in the discussion of models of subcortical participation in language below.

# Neuroanatomical models of subcortical participation in language

In recent years a number of different theories regarding subcortical functions in language have been proposed. Three theories, in particular, appear to have been the subject of most discussion in the literature. These include the model proposed by Alexander et al. (1987), that proposed by Crosson (1985) and finally, the theory put forward by Wallesch and Papagno (1988). The model proposed by Alexander et al. (1987) suggests only a minimal role for the striatum in language. According to their theory, aphasia associated with subcortical lesions is caused primarily by disruption of cortico-cortical connections as they traverse the subcortical region. In contrast the models proposed by Crosson (1985) and Wallesch and Papagno (1988) both attribute specific language functions to the various subcortical structures. In particular, these latter two models propose that interaction between the cortex, basal ganglia and thalamus is important for correct, efficient language production.

### Model 1: Alexander et al. (1987)

This model, referred to by Crosson (1992) as the 'subcortical pathway model' stresses the importance of white matter pathways to language function and downplays the role of structures such as the putamen, caudate nucleus and globus pallidus. Alexander et al. (1987) based their theory on their observation that isolated cerebrovascular lesions in the striatum caused only minimal disruption to normal language, their subjects exhibiting, at most, only mild word-finding difficulty or hesitancy in verbal output.

They accounted for the observed language disturbance after larger striatal lesions by the fact that subcortical vascular lesions, in the majority of cases, almost always involve white matter pathways as well as the basal ganglia. They asserted that, in the case of non-thalamic subcortical lesions, it is the interruption of cortico-cortical pathways traversing subcortical space that is the factor causing the language dysfunction. The Alexander et al. (1987) model therefore clearly focuses attention on the subcortical white matter pathways of the dominant hemisphere as important to language. This proposition would seem quite reasonable, since these pathways are the means by which the various components of the language system communicate with one another. The white matter pathways implicated in language include the medial subcallosal fasciculus which carries fibres from the mesial frontal cortex (supplementary motor area and anterior cingulate gyrus) to the caudate nucleus and may be involved in the initiation of language and speech. Other subcortical pathways connect one cortical area with another, such as the connections between the supplementary motor area and Broca's area, or the connections between the posterior and anterior language areas which are contained in the arcuate fasciculus. The subcortical white matter also carries other pathways that have been implicated in language, including cortico-thalamic connections, thalamo-cortical connections, cortico-striatal pathways (e.g. between the posterior/language cortex and the head of the caudate nucleus), striato-pallidal connections and pallido-thalamic connections.

## Model 2: Crosson (1985)

Crosson (1985) incorporated Ojemann's (1976) activating role of the subcortical structures within a neuroanatomically based model of language processing. He developed a model which not only considers cortico-cortical connections but includes the dynamic interrelationships between the cortex, basal ganglia and the thalamus and accounts for the way information flows between these structures in the production of language. In Crosson's (1985) model two cortical language areas are described, including an anterior and posterior centre. Language formulation (e.g. conceptual, wordfinding and syntactic processes), motor programming and decoding of complex grammar are regarded as functions of the anterior language centre situated in the frontal cortex. The posterior language centre is located in the temporo-parietal cortex and is involved in decoding semantic and phonological information. The anterior and posterior centres communicate with each other via the arcuate fasciculus which is involved in phonological processing. Crosson (1985) suggested that the temporo-parietal structures, which are responsible for phonemic discrimination, monitor the motor programming of language through the arcuate fasciculus and determine whether the motor programme conforms to the desired phonological pattern. Hence, a lesion in the arcuate fasciculus has traditionally been thought to result in conduction aphasia characterised by impaired repetition abilities and the presence of phonemic paraphasias in spontaneous speech (Goodglass and Kaplan, 1983).

In his model, Crosson (1985) proposed that the thalamus acts to activate or arouse the cortex and monitor the semantic content of language encoded by the anterior language area. Direct and indirect fibres connect the brainstem reticular formation, which is associated with waking mechanisms (Guyton, 1981), and the ventral anterior nucleus of the thalamus. These reticulo-thalamic fibres transfer alerting information to the frontal cortex via the anterior limb of the internal capsule. The ventral anterior nucleus selectively excites the anterior language zones of the frontal cortex and provides the appropriate level of cortical activation for language production. Crosson (1985) proposed that, if cortical excitation remains too high, extraneous information enters the encoder and motor programmer for production. For example, over excitation of the cortex may result in the production of extraneous paraphasic errors (Kennedy and Murdoch, 1989). In contrast, with low cortical tone, language formulation may be inefficient, dysfluent, or may not occur spontaneously at all (Damasio et al., 1982).

According to the model, reciprocal connections between the thalamus and the cortex provide a feedback loop enabling preverbal semantic monitoring to occur (Crosson, 1985). The thalamus not only acts to alert the cortex but also enables the temporo-parietal areas of the cortex to monitor the encoding of language carried out in the anterior language centre before it is produced. Language formulated in the anterior language centre is transmitted via a cortico-thalamo-cortical pathway to the posterior temporo-parietal language centre which decodes and checks the semantic input. The most probable pathway for this information transfer from the anterior to posterior language centres is via connections with the ventral anterior thalamus and the pulvinar. In order for the message to be modified, the semantic information is then conveyed via the same pathway back to the anterior cortex to be corrected and then produced as speech.

Crosson (1985) proposed that the basal ganglia may be involved in two mechanisms which influence language production by integrating inputs from the cortex and subsequently influencing thalamic and ultimately cortical mechanisms. These processes are as follows: the basal ganglia (in particular the global pallidus) may influence tone in the anterior cortical language areas by regulating the flow of excitatory impulses from the ventral anterior thalamus; also, the basal ganglia (caudate nucleus) may act as a motor release mechanism that allows language segments to be 'motor programmed' after semantic monitoring has taken place. As part of his model, Crosson (1985) suggested that the posterior language decoder and anterior language formulator are located in close proximity to a motor programmer. In order for a language segment to be released, once it has been monitored, the integrity of the basal ganglia is necessary to perform a motor release function. Under the control of the temporo-parietal cortex the basal ganglia act as a motor release mechanism permitting language segments to be released at the appropriate time. The putamen and caudate nucleus of the basal ganglia receive fibres from various regions of the cerebral cortex but do not send fibres directly to the cortex. Therefore, information is transferred out via the globus pallidus, which indirectly influences the cortex through connections with the ventral anterior nuclei of the thalamus. On the basis of anatomical findings, Crosson (1985) attributed an indirect function of modifying cortical tonic activity to the basal ganglia. He suggested that the globus pallidus, by inhibition, regulates the amount of excitatory neural impulses flowing from the ventral anterior thalamus. The ventral anterior thalamus, in turn, activates the cortical language centres for language production.

In normal semantic verification of language, Crosson (1985) suggested that inhibitory influences from the temporo-parietal cortex (decoded as language segments requiring modification) prevent language segments from being released as speech. The posterior language cortex exerts a negative influence on the head of the caudate nucleus which disinhibits the globus pallidus, which in turn leads to increased inhibition of the thalamus and decreased excitation of the anterior language cortex, with the consequence that no speech is produced. Once the semantic information is monitored as correct, the temporo-parietal cortex acts to temporarily inhibit pallidal mechanisms, thereby releasing the ventral anterior thalamic nuclei from pallidal inhibition. The thalamus subsequently increases its excitation to the anterior cortical mechanisms, thus allowing the release of a semantically verified language segment for motor programming.

Crosson (1985) proposed that lesions in the thalamus may disrupt arousal of the cortex and disturb the process of preverbal semantic monitoring. The frequent loss of spontaneous speech following thalamic lesions (Jonas, 1982) may be due to the interruption of excitatory input from the thalamus to the cortex. Thalamic lesions may interrupt the transfer of information between the anterior and posterior language centres, and thus disrupt preverbal semantic monitoring. The presence of poorly monitored semantic content of language, characterised by the production of semantic paraphasias following thalamic lesions (Alexander and LoVerme, 1980; Bogousslavsky et al., 1988; Kennedy and

Murdoch, 1989), can be explained by disturbed preverbal semantic monitoring. Dysfluent speech may occur after disruption of thalamo-cortical fibres lying in the anterior limb of the internal capsule (Damasio et al., 1982). A lesion interrupting communication between the ventral anterior nucleus of the thalamus and the anterior language centre may decrease the level of cortical excitation from the thalamus and inhibit language formulation in the anterior language centre. Subjects with lesions in the subcortical white matter pathways required for preverbal semantic monitoring would be expected to present with limited verbal output and relatively intact comprehension abilities. According to Crosson's (1985) model this language pattern occurs because the decoding mechanism remains intact but the monitoring of semantic information is disrupted. Repetition would also remain intact due to reliance on intact phonological pathways in the arcuate fasciculus (Bogousslavsky et al., 1988; Mateer and Ojemann, 1983; Tuszynski and Petito, 1988).

On the basis of this model, it can be predicted that lesions in the globus pallidus lead to reduced inhibition of the ventral anterior nucleus of the thalamus and subsequent disinhibition of tonic activity of the cortex. The over-excitation of the cortex by the thalamus allows extraneous information to enter the encoding language centre and fluent extraneous language characteristics result (e.g. semantic para-phasias). A study by Naeser et al. (1982) also described subjects with a fluent type of aphasia following capsular-putaminal lesions with anterior white matter extensions. The subjects in this group exhibited aphasic characteristics including semantic paraphasias.

Crosson (1985) suggested that lesions in the caudate nucleus lead to a non-fluent output due to disinhibition of the globus pallidus, inhibi-tion of the ventral anterior nucleus and a decrease in tonic activation of the anterior language zone. These non-fluent characteristics of aphasia have been found in subjects with capsular-putaminal lesions with poste-rior white matter extensions (Naeser et al., 1982).

Subcortical pathway disruption may influence the tonic activity of the cortex and result in fluent or non-fluent speech production (Crosson, 1985). For example, lesions in striato-pallidal fibres may lead to disinhi-bition of the globus pallidus, subsequently increase inhibitory influence on the ventral anterior nucleus of the thalamus and decrease cortical activation in the anterior language centre resulting in a paucity of spon-taneous speech and dysfluency once speech is initiated. Lesions in pallido-thalamic fibres, however, may result in a reduced inhibitory influence of the globus pallidus on the ventral anterior nucleus of the thalamus, leading to increased level of excitation in the anterior language area and fluent aphasic characteristics, including the presence of extraneous speech and semantic paraphasias in conversation.

Interference in the subcortical pathways in close proximity with the caudate nucleus connecting the temporo-parietal posterior language centre with the caudate nucleus may result in inappropriate disinhibition of the caudate nucleus. In turn, disinhibition of the caudate nucleus may lead to increased inhibition of the globus pallidus, excitation of the thalamus and an increased level of activation of the anterior language cortex. Increased excitation of the cortex may allow the release of extraneous, poorly monitored language for motor programming, reflecting a fluent type of aphasia. In contrast, subjects with lesions interrupting fronto-caudate fibres, pathways used to terminate utterances in normal speech production, may exhibit a non-fluent aphasic characteristic such as perseveration. Naeser et al. (1982) described a group of subjects with capsular-putaminal lesions with anterior and posterior white matter extensions who presented with a global type of aphasia including perseverative speech production. The subject discussed by Gordon (1985) presented with fronto-caudate lesions and exhibited a non-fluent Broca's type of aphasia.

Crosson (1985) has described a non-fluent type of aphasia following a lesion in the anterior limb of the internal capsule. Extensive lesions in the anterior limb of the internal capsule may disrupt efferent corticostriatal connections, such as the fronto-caudate pathways as well as reciprocal thalamo-cortical pathways, and act to disconnect the cortex from the caudate nucleus and the putamen. As a result of this disconnection the cortex is unable to receive information from the subcortical structures and vice versa. Therefore, there is decreased excitation of the anterior language cortex responsible for language formulation and motor programming so that subjects with lesions in the anterior limb of the internal capsule have difficulty initiating spontaneous speech (Damasio et al., 1982).

It is important to note that the clinical presentations of subjects following lesions in specific subcortical pathways and structures outlined above are largely speculative, being based on predicted language outcomes according to the author's interpretation of Crosson's (1985) model. According to this model, semantic problems in the form of verbal paraphasic errors could result from lesions in either the thalamus or basal ganglia. In agreement with this prediction, a number of authors have reported the occurrence of semantic paraphasias in association with both thalamic (Alexander and LoVerme, 1980; Cappa and Vignolo, 1979) and basal ganglia (Damasio et al., 1982; Wallesch, 1985) lesions. Also consistent with the model, a number of studies (Damasio et al., 1982; Naeser et al.,1982) have found that destruction of the anterior limb of the internal capsule produces dysfluent but often grammatical language.

The model proposed by Crosson (1985) has also been subjected to some criticism. Kennedy and Murdoch (1989) suggested that Crosson's evidence for the existence of a process 'preverbal semantic monitoring' was scant, and that some aspects of the aphasic disturbances observed in the subjects with subcortical lesions in their study could not be readily accounted for by the model (e.g. comprehension deficits, no response errors in naming). Furthermore, Robin and Schienberg (1990) indicated that Crosson's model could not account for the presence of neologisms in the speech of their thalamic aphasics. Wallesch and Papagno (1988) were also critical of Crosson's (1985) model, but from a more anatomical/physiological perspective. These latter authors advocated that Crosson's (1985) model is too localisationist and that the important linguistic operation of sentence assembly does not necessarily occur in the left frontal area of the cortex and that formulation of sentences or propositions cannot be localised in the cortex. Wallesch and Papagno (1988) also objected to Crosson's (1985) proposed role of the thalamus in language processing in which non-specific thalamic nuclei perform very specific functions by connecting anterior and posterior language zones. They pointed out that Crosson (1985) assumed that the ventral anterior nucleus of the thalamus performs two different functions and acts in two opposite directions. The ventral thalamus (according to Crosson, 1985) acts to transfer linguistic information bidirectionally between frontal and temporo-parietal cortical language areas, simultaneously selectively distributing excitatory influences from the reticular formation to the cortex. This multiple function theory for one single thalamic nucleus was regarded as inadequate by Wallesch and Papagno (1988). One final problem with Crosson's (1985) model is that it predicts the presence of an inhibitory neurotransmitter substance between the temporo-parietal cortex and the dominant caudate nucleus (Crosson, 1992). However, there is evidence available to suggest that the transmitter is glutamate, an excitatory transmitter (Koscis, Sugimori and Kitai, 1977).

Crosson's (1985) model was the subject of a revision by Crosson and Early (1990; cited in Crosson, 1992). Consistent with the criticism mounted by Wallesch and Papagno (1988), they agreed that, although the mechanisms proposed by the 1985 model were viable, the neuroanatomical substrates of the model required revision (Crosson, 1992). Rather than the cortico-striato-pallido-thalamo-cortical loop being involved in both tonic arousal of the frontal cortex and the response-release mechanism, they suggested that the loop was involved in only the latter function. They proposed that the tonic arousal mechanism operates from the thalamic intralaminar nuclei (which receive input from the midbrain reticular formation) directly to the frontal cortex. Although the fibres passing from the thalamic intralaminar nuclei to the frontal cortex do so via the ventral anterior nucleus of the thalamus, as suggested by Jones (1985), they do so without giving off collaterals to the ventral anterior nucleus. According to Crosson (1992), the revised model is more consistent with the effects of thalamic infarction on language documented by several studies (Bogousslavsky et al., 1988; Graff-Radford et al., 1984) in that although the 1985 model predicts decreased fluency associated with lesions involving the ventral anterior nucleus, characteristics of both fluent and non-fluent output have been reported. In addition, the revised model fits better with reports that the cortico-striatal neurotransmitter is excitatory in nature (Kocsis et al., 1977) and is more consistent with thalamic neuroanatomy as reported by Jones (1985).

### Model 3: Wallesch and Papagno (1988)

Wallesch and Papagno (1988) proposed a model of subcortical participation in language that attributes an even greater role for the striatum than that proposed by Crosson (1985). In many ways, therefore, their model is at the opposite end of the spectrum from the minimal participation role assigned to the striatum in the model of Alexander et al.(1987). Wallesch and Papagno's (1988) model incorporates elements of Crosson's (1985) language processing model and also Ojemann's (1976) language specific, cortically alerting function of the thalamus. Counter to Crosson's (1985) more localisationist view, however, Wallesch and Papagno (1988) suggested that language functions are not discretely represented in one single location in the cortex. They indicated that the basic functional unit of the cortex is the 'module' and that these modules allow for parallel processing of information (i.e. in line with the rising popularity of distributed-network theories of language processing). The module is held to be defined by its thalamic afferent, and as such the thalamus is in a position to modify cortical function.

According to Wallesch and Papagno's (1988) model, the cortico-striato-pallido-thalamo-cortical loop forms the anatomical basis of subcortical participation in language. They suggested that this loop is involved in monitoring and selecting from multiple lexical alternatives originating in the posterior language cortex and transmitted forward to the anterior cortex in a modular fashion. In particular they described a frontal lobe system in which the head of the caudate nucleus, the globus pallidus and the ventral thalamus are integrated to influence the frontal cortex. In communication, according to their model, these subcortical structures together are involved in response selection by gating among a number of possible lexical alternatives generated in the posterior cortex. That is, efferent modules work both in parallel and in competition and the thalamus, under the influence of the basal ganglia, works to integrate and/or gate the information, choose the desired response and then transmit features of a central command to the frontal cortex. To some extent, therefore, their model puts the striatum in a superordinate position with respect to the cerebral cortex, in that it regulates which among several cortically generated lexical alternatives are expressed. Wallesch and

Papagno's (1988) model, therefore, requires the striatum to have a greater information processing capability than required by Crosson's (1985) model, in which the cortico-striato-pallido-thalamo-cortical loop plays more of a regulatory role vis-a-vis the cortex.

In Wallesch and Papagno's (1988) model of language processing, the cortex, within each module, transmits relevant information regarding the task (e.g. situational constraints and volitional goal directed demands) to the striatum via cortico-striatal fibres. The striatum then acts to provide possible responses fitting the criteria stipulated by the cortex, that is, the striatum integrates and organises the incoming cortical information. Each module provides an alternative which is transmitted to the thalamus via the globus pallidus, but only one response is released by the thalamus to be produced by the frontal cortex. The globus pallidus controls and modulates by inhibition of the thalamus via pallido-thalamic fibres. Therefore, inhibition of the thalamus causes closure of the thalamic gate, which decreases the number of inhibitory messages travelling to the frontal cortex (premotor) and leads to production of the desired response. In reactive language (e.g. repetition), where all the responses produced by different modules are the same, there is no competition, the gating response is not effective and the language segment is released. If there is competition, however, only one module inhibits the thalamus, closes the thalamic gate and releases the cortex from inhibition so that a response is released. Other extraneous responses are not released because the global pallidus acts to disinhibit the thalamus in the remaining modules.

Wallesch and Papagno (1988) suggested that the striatum may involve both internal and efferent excitatory mechanisms. Therefore, striatal lesions could result in either inhibitory and disinhibitory effects of the globus pallidus which, in turn, influence the ventral thalamus and lead to diverse language deficits. Similarly, it is predicted from Wallesch and Papagno's (1988) model that subjects with lesions disrupting striato-pallidal pathways may result in diverse language deficits.

On the basis of their model, Wallesch and Papagno (1988) predicted that lesions in the globus pallidus lead to the inability of the globus pallidus to inhibit the ventral thalamus. Thus, the thalamus is disinhibited so that the thalamic gate is opened, the cortex is inhibited and no language is produced. Clinical evidence which supports this process of gating is found in the presence of transcortical motor type aphasia following pallidal lesions (Brunner et al., 1982; Damasio et al., 1982). The inhibitory effect of the thalamus on the cortex unimpeded explains characteristics of subcortical aphasia such as the inability to initiate conversation as well as the production of dysfluent speech once initiated.

The presence of relatively preserved morphosyntactical operations, repetition and naming abilities reported in subcortical aphasia have also been explained by Wallesch and Papagno (1988) in terms of 'degrees of freedom'. Wallesch and Papagno (1988) suggested that, due to the presence of a parallel system, even with pallidal lesions, a semantically and syntactically appropriate response eventually will be produced on language tasks with restricted degrees of freedom (e.g. repetition). Language evoked by external stimulation, such as repetition, has restricted degrees of freedom. That is, there are a limited number of responses which can be formulated by the different modules. Therefore, even if thalamic gating is not accurate, all parallel modules generate the same response and there is no competition. Limited degrees of freedom are also evident in morphosyntactical operations where rules restrict possible alternatives such as the order of words in a sentence and which verb form to use in a certain linguistic environment. Conversely, the lexical content in spontaneous speech production and the generation of names on a word fluency task allow many degrees of freedom. Many more appropriate responses can fit the criteria proposed by the cortex. Competing parallel options must be integrated and responses selected by the subcortical circuitry system. Wallesch and Papagno (1988) found that those tasks with more degrees of freedom were more severely affected after lesions in the subcortex. Other researchers have also described subjects, following subcortical CVAs, exhibiting disrupted spontaneous speech while maintaining relatively preserved syntactic, repetition and naming abilities (Alexander and LoVerme, 1980; Damasio et al., 1982; Naeser et al., 1982).

Naeser et al. (1982) reported on a group of subjects with capsular/putaminal lesions with anterior superior white matter extensions who presented with non-fluent grammatical language production. In Damasio et al.'s (1982) study, a subject presented with a lesion extending into the caudate nucleus, the putamen and the surrounding white matter. This subject exhibited non-fluent language characteristics but performed normally on tasks with low degrees of freedom (e.g. repetition). Based on the model proposed by Wallesch and Papagno (1988), it would be predicted that similar non-fluent type aphasia resulting from pallidal lesions would also result from a lesion in pallido-thalamic fibres. Disruption of these pathways may also lead to disinhibition of the thalamus and opening of the thalamic gate, allowing inhibitory messages to reach the frontal cortex and prevent language production.

The production of semantic paraphasias evident in subcortical aphasia (Alexander and LoVerme, 1980; Gorelick et al., 1984; Kennedy and Murdoch, 1989; Wallesch, 1985) may be explained by a disrupted gating mechanism in Wallesch and Papagno's (1988) model. Lesions in the thalamus may lead to the release of inappropriate, poorly monitored responses by the frontal cortex. The thalamus may receive inhibitory input from the globus pallidus in order to produce a response, but due to the thalamic lesion, all gates in the thalamus are permanently closed. The cortex is disinhibited and all parallel circuits may arrive at the cortex for a response. The first response completing the circuit and reaching the cortex will be produced rather than the correct response. Similarly, it is speculated that thalamo-cortical fibre lesions will disconnect the thalamus from the cortex so that information released by the thalamus is unable to reach the frontal cortex for production. This disconnection is clearly evident in the subcortical aphasic characteristic of paucity of spontaneous speech.

Researchers have proposed that a modular system allows combinations and recombinations of inputs, thus presenting an adaptive or plastic mechanism for information processing (Goldman-Rakic, 1984). Wallesch and Papagno (1988) have suggested that language functions in chronic subcortical conditions (e.g. Parkinson's disease) may be spared due to functional plasticity of the cortico-subcortical system. Direct links, such as the cortico-cortical pathways, and bypasses, such as the fronto-thalamo-cortical pathway, may enable function reorganisation. Indeed, slow progression of chronic diseases may allow time for pathways to reorganise. The complex integrative circuitry of the basal ganglia, including internal excitatory and inhibitory mechanisms, may also account for the clinical diversity of language disorders resulting from lesions in the subcortical structures and their pathways (Wallesch and Papagno, 1988).

In summary, Wallesch and his colleagues (1983, 1985, 1988) proposed that, under the control of the frontal cortex, the basal ganglia and the thalamus are responsible for integrating information and selecting an appropriate response from a number of parallel choices. Lesions in the structures and pathways of this parallel system account for the clinical characteristics of subcortical aphasia including poor initiation of speech (Alexander and LoVerme, 1980), reduced word fluency (Kennedy and Murdoch, 1989), semantic paraphasias (Wallesch, 1985), intact syntax (Jonas, 1982) and relatively preserved repetition abilities (Alexander and LoVerme, 1980). According to Wallesch and his colleagues (1983, 1985, 1988), lesions in the deep nuclei mostly affect lexical functions and result in anomia and semantic paraphasias. They suggest that the presence of neologisms and jargon associated with disturbed processing and wordfinding deficits depends on the degrees of freedom which are potentially available to the subject in any given situation (e.g. word finding in spontaneous speech versus confrontation naming).

According to Wallesch and Papagno's (1988) parallel processing model, language processing can only take place if communication links between cortical and subcortical structures, and between the subcortical structures themselves (via white matter pathways) are preserved. Cortico-striatal tracts contain fibres connecting the precentral motor cortex with the putamen (Tanridag and Krishner, 1987), and the association areas of the prefrontal, temporal and parietal cortex primarily with the caudate nucleus (Goldman-Rakic, 1984). Hence, lesions in these tracts would interrupt cortico-subcortical information transfer and disrupt language production. A lesion interrupting striato-pallidal connections is likely to disrupt lexical information travelling from the striatum to the globus pallidus so that incomplete signals are transmitted to the thalamus.

## Limitations of models of subcortical participation in language

As pointed out by Crosson (1992), a major problem with all neuroanatomical models of subcortical participation in language proposed to date is the difficulty in verifying their accuracy given the inherent inadequacies of currently available neuro-imaging techniques. The majority of the evidence linking subcortical lesions to the occurrence of aphasia reported in the literature so far has come from studies based on CT localisation of lesion sites. Unfortunately, the extent of impairment of structure and function cannot be exactly defined on the basis of CT. For instance, CT may miss small infarctions under 5 mm in diameter (Wodarz, 1980), and some lesions that appear to involve only subcortical structures on CT have been shown to involve the cortex as well with MRI (DeWitt et al., 1985). It has been suggested, therefore, that CT may be inadequate to define the actual extent of brain lesions and consequently, the aphasia documented in association with subcortical lesions defined by CT may be due to unidentified, small structural lesions involving the cortex. Although language problems have been documented in association with subcortical lesions defined by MRI (Murdoch et al., 1991), both CT and MRI are unable to detect partial selective loss of neurones in the cortex (Lassen, Olsen, Hojgaard and Skriver, 1983). As support for the concept that subcortical structures participate in language, however, a number of recent clinico-anatomical reports have shown that aphasia may be associated with subcortical lesions without any macroscopic or microscopic cortical abnormality (Barat et al., 1981; Bogousslavsky et al., 1988; Tuszynski and Petito, 1988).

In addition to inadequacies of current lesion localisation methods, another problem in seeking a causal relationship between subcortical lesions identified by CT or MRI and aphasia is that subcortical lesions may produce remote or distance effects on the cerebral cortex which may interfere with cortical functioning and thereby produce neurobehavioural problems. These distance effects include a depression of cortical metabolism (Baron et al., 1986; Metter et al., 1983, 1986) and a reduction in cortical blood flow (Perani et al., 1987; Skyhoj-Olsen, Bruhn and Oberg, 1986; Weinrich et al., 1987). Some authors (e.g. Skyhoj-Olsen et al., 1986) believe that these distance effects are responsible for the production of language deficits seen in association with subcortical lesions rather than these deficits being the direct outcome of the subcortical lesions. At present most authors agree, however, that distance effects, including metabolic abnormalities and reduced blood flow in the cortex following subcortical damage are best explained in terms of diaschisis, i.e. reduced functional activity due to deprivation from afferent input as a result of disconnection of two brain regions (Cappa and Vallar, 1992; Kushner et al., 1987). Clearly, this interpretation of distance effects as resulting from diaschisis is based on the existence of neural networks which involve both the cortex and subcortical structures (Cappa and Vallar, 1992). That subcortical lesions associated with a language disorder (subcortical aphasia) can cause alterations in cortical metabolism and cortical regional cerebral blood flow by disconnecting subcortical structures such as the striatum and thalamus from the cerebral cortex suggests that the neural substrate of the language disorder itself is disruption of complex neural circuits that involve the primary area of structural damage as well as other connected but distant brain regions.

## Conclusions

Although the study of language disorders in subjects with apparent subcortical lesions has led to the development of several theories regarding subcortical language processing, the role of structures such as the thalamus and basal ganglia in language remains controversial. In particular, the participation of the basal ganglia in language remains unclear. Although some authors have suggested that the basal ganglia are only minimally involved in language (e.g. Alexander et al., 1987), anatomical, physiological and clinical evidence suggests that the basal ganglia and thalamus form essential parts of neural networks that subserve language. Most recent models of subcortical participation in language (e.g. Crosson, 1985; Crosson and Early, 1990; Wallesch and Papagno, 1988) propose that cortico-striato-pallido-thalamo-cortical loops are involved in language.

Given their limitations in accurate localisation of subcortical lesion sites, however, it is unlikely that clinico-anatomical studies based on either CT or MRI will further elucidate the role of various subcortical structures in language. Consequently, rather than pursuing this line of research further, future studies should apply functional brain imaging methods such as positron emission tomography (PET) and single photon emission computed tomography (SPECT) to the study of normal subjects along the lines of studies reported by Petersen et al. (1988). Perhaps it is only by turning our attention away from the study of brain impaired subjects and applying these new technologies to individuals with normal language that further illumination of the role of subcortical structures in language will be obtained.

# References

Alexander, G.E. and Crutcher, M.D. (1990). Functional architecture of basal ganglia circuits: Neural substrates of parallel processing. *Trends in Neuroscience*, **13**, 266–271.

Alexander, G.E. and LoVerme, S.R. (1980). Aphasia after left hemisphere intracerebral haemorrhage. *Neurology*, **30**, 1193–1202.

Alexander, G.E., DeLong, M.R. and Strick, P.L. (1986). Parallel organisation of functionally segregated circuits linking basal ganglia and cortex. *Annual Review of Neuroscience*, **9**, 357–381.

Alexander, G.E., Naeser, M.A. and Palumbo, C.L. (1987). Correlations of subcortical CT lesions sites and aphasia profiles. *Brain*, **110**, 961–991.

Aten, J.L., White, B.J. and Pribram, H.W. (1982). Linguistic and behavioural deficits following thalamic haemorrhage. In R.H. Brookshire (Ed.) *Clinical Aphasiology: Conference Proceedings*, pp. 119–128. Minneapolis MN: BRK.

Barat, M., Mazaux, J.M., Bioulac, B., Giroire, J.M., Vital, C. and Arne, L. (1981). Troubles due langage de type aphasique et lesions putamino-caudees. *Revue Neurologique*, **137**, 343–356.

Baron, J.C.D., Antona, R., Pantano, P., Serdaru, M., Samson, Y. and Bouser, M.G. (1986). Effects of thalamic stroke on energy metabolism of the cerebral cortex: A positron tomography study in man. *Brain*, **119**, 1243–1259.

Bogousslavsky, J., Regli, F. and Uske, A. (1988). Thalamic infarcts: Clinical syndromes, aetiology and prognosis. *Neurology*, **38**, 837–848.

Brunner, R.J., Kornhuber, H.H., Seemuller, E., Suger, G. and Wallesch, C.W. (1982). Basal ganglia participation in language pathology. *Brain and Language*, **16**, 281–299.

Bruyn, R.P.M. (1989). Thalamic aphasia: A conceptual critique. *Journal of Neurology*, **236**, 21–25.

Cappa, S.F. and Vallar, G. (1992). Neuropsychological disorders after subcortical lesions: Implications for neural models of language and spatial attention. In G. Valler, S.F. Cappa and C.W. Wallesch (Eds) *Neuropsychological Disorders Associated with Subcortical Lesions*. New York: Oxford University Press.

Cappa, S.F. and Vignolo, L.A. (1979). Transcortical features of aphasia following left thalamic haemorrhage. *Cortex*, **15**, 121–130.

Cappa, S.F., Cavallotti, G., Guidotti, M., Papagno, C. and Vignolo, L.A. (1983). Subcortical aphasia: Two clinical–CT correlation studies. *Cortex*, **19**, 227–241.

Chesson, A.L. (1983). Aphasia following a right thalamic haemorrhage. *Brain and Language*, **19**, 306–316.

Crosson, B. (1985). Subcortical functions in language: A working model. *Brain and Language*, **25**, 257–292.

Crosson, B. (1992). *Subcortical Functions in Language and Memory*. New York: The Guilford Press.

Crosson, B. and Early, T.S. (1990). A theory of subcortical functions in language: Current status. Cited in Crosson, 1992, p. 132.

Damasio, A.R., Damasio, H., Rizzo, M., Varney, N. and Gersh, F. (1982). Aphasia with nonhaemorrhagic lesions in the basal ganglia and internal capsule. *Archives of Neurology*, **39**, 15–20.

DeWitt, L.D., Grek, A.J., Buonanno, F.S., Levine, D.N. and Kistler, J.P. (1985). MRI and the study of aphasia. *Neurology*, **35**, 861–865.

Fedio, P. and Van Buren, J.M. (1975). Memory and perceptual deficits during electrical stimulation in the left and right thalamus and parietal subcortex. *Brain and Language*, **2**, 78–100.

Goldman-Rakic, P.S. (1984). Modular organisation of the prefrontal cortex. *Trends in Neuroscience*, **7**, 419–424.

Goodglass, H. and Kaplan, E. (1983). Boston diagnostic aphasia examination. In H. Goodglass and E. Kaplan (Eds) *The Assessment of Aphasia and Related Disorders*, 2nd edn. Philadelphia: Lea & Febiger.

Gordon, W.P. (1985). Neuropsychologic assessment of aphasia. In J.K. Darby, *Speech and Language Evaluation in Neurology: Adult Disorders*, pp. 161–196. Orlando: Grune & Stratton.

Gorelick, P.B., Hier, D.B., Benevento, L., Levitt, S. and Tan, W. (1984). Aphasia after left thalamic infarction. *Archives of Neurology*, **41**, 1296–1298.

Graff-Radford, N.R., Eslinger, P.J., Damasio, A.R. and Yamada, T. (1984). Nonhaemorrhagic infarction of the thalamus: Behaviour, anatomic and physiological correlates. *Neurology*, **34**, 14–23.

Guyton, A.C. (1981). *Textbook of Medical Physiology*, 6th edn. Philadelphia: Saunders.

Jonas, S. (1982). The thalamus and aphasia, including transcortical aphasia: A review. *Journal of Communication Disorders*, **15**, 31–41.

Jones, E.G. (1985). *The Thalamus*. New York: Plenum Press.

Kennedy, M. and Murdoch, B.E. (1989). Speech and language disorders subsequent to subcortical vascular lesions. *Aphasiology*, **3**, 221–247.

Kennedy, M. and Murdoch, B.E. (1993). Chronic aphasia subsequent to striatocapsular and thalamic lesions in the left hemisphere. *Brain and Language*, **44**, 284–295.

Kocsis, J.D., Sugimori, M. and Kitai, S.T. (1977). Convergence of excitatory synaptic inputs to caudate spiny neurons. *Brain Research*, **124**, 403–413.

Kushner, M.J., Reivich, M., Fieschi, C., Silver, F., Chawluk, J., Rosen, M., Greenberg, J., Burke, A. and Alavi, A. (1987). Metabolic and clinical correlates of acute ischaemic infarction. *Neurology*, **37**, 1103–1110.

Lassen, N.A., Olsen, T., Hojgaard, K. and Skriver, E. (1983). Incomplete infarction: A CT–negative irreversible ischaemic brain lesion. *Journal of Cerebral Blood Flow and Metabolism*, **3**, (Suppl. 1), 602–603.

Lichtheim, L. (1885). On aphasia. *Brain*, **7**, 433–484.

Luria, A.R. (1977). On quasi–aphasic speech disturbances in lesions of the deep structure of the brain. *Brain and Language*, **4**, 432–459.

Mateer, C.A. and Ojemann, G.A. (1983). Thalamic mechanisms in language and memory. In S.J. Segalowitz (Ed.) *Language Functions and Brain Organization*, pp.171–191. New York: Academic Press.

McFarling, D., Rothi, L.J. and Heilman, K.M. (1982). Transcortical aphasia from ischaemic infarcts of the thalamus. A report of two cases. *Journal of Neurology, Neurosurgery, and Psychiatry*, **45**, 107–112.

Mesulam, M.M. (1981). A cortical network for directed attention and unilateral neglect. *Annals of Neurology*, **10**, 309–325.

Metter, E.J., Riege, W.R., Hanson, W.R., Kuhl, D.E., Phelps, M.E., Squire, L.R., Wasterlain, C.G. and Benson, D.F. (1983). Comparison of metabolic rates, language and memory in subcortical aphasias. *Brain and Language*, **19**, 33–47.

Metter, E.J., Jackson, C., Kempler, D., Rieger, W.H., Hanson, W.R., Mazziotta, J.C. and Phelps, M.E. (1986). Left hemisphere intracerebral haemorrhages studied by (F-18)- flurodeoxyglucose PET. *Neurology*, **36**, 1115–1162.

Metter, E.J., Riege, W.R., Hanson, W.R., Jackson, C.A., Kempler, D. and Van Lancker, D. (1988). Subcortical structures in aphasia: Analysis based on (F-18)-flurodeoxyglucose positron emission tomography and computed tomography. *Archives of Neurology*, **45**, 1229–1234.

Mohr, J.P., Watters, W.C. and Duncan, G.W. (1975). Thalamic haemorrhage and aphasia. *Brain and Language*, **2**, 3–17.

Murdoch, B.E. (1987). Aphasia following right thalamic hemorrhage in a dextral. *Journal of Communication Disorders*, **20**, 459–468.

Murdoch, B.E., Kennedy, M., McCallum, W. and Siddle, K.J. (1991). Persistent aphasia following a purely subcortical lesion: A magnetic resonance imaging study. *Aphasiology*, **5**, 183–197.

Naeser, M.A., Alexander, M.P., Helm-Estabrooks, N., Levine, H.L., Laughlin, S.A. and Geschwind, N. (1982). Aphasia with predominantly subcortical lesion sites: Description of three capsular/putaminal aphasia syndromes. *Archives of Neurology*, **39**, 2–14.

Naeser, M.A., Palumbo, C.L., Helm-Estabrooks, N., Stiassny-Eder, D. and Albert, M.L. (1989). Severe nonfluency in aphasia: Role of the medial subcallosal fasciculus and other white matter pathways in recovery of spontaneous speech. *Brain*, **112**, 1–38.

Ojemann, G.A. (1975). Language and the thalamus: Object naming and recall during and after thalamic stimulation. *Brain and Language*, **2**, 101–120.

Ojemann, G.A. (1976). Subcortical language mechanisms. In H. Whitaker and H.A. Whitaker (Eds), *Studies in Neurolinguistics*, pp. 103–138. New York: Academic Press.

Ojemann, G.A. (1977). Asymmetric function of the thalamus in man. *Annals of the New York Academy of Science*, **299**, 380–396.

Ojemann, G.A. and Ward, A.A. (1971). Speech representation in ventrolateral thalamus. *Brain*, **26**, 669–680.

Penfield, W. and Roberts, L. (1959). *Speech and Brain Mechanisms*. Princeton: Princeton University Press.

Perani, D., Vallar, G., Cappa, S., Messa, C. and Fazio, F. (1987). Aphasia and neglect after subcortical stroke: A clinical/cerebral perfusion correlation study. *Brain*, **110**, 1211–1229.

Petersen, S.E., Fox, P.T., Posner, M.I., Mintum, M. and Raichle, M.E. (1988). Positron emission tomographic studies of the cortical anatomy of single-word processing. *Nature*, **331**, 585–589.

Riklan, M. and Cooper, I.S. (1975). Psychometric studies of verbal functions following thalamic lesions in humans. *Brain and Language*, **2**, 45–64.

Riklan, M. and Levita, E. (1970). Psychological studies of thalamic lesions in humans. *Journal of Nervous and Mental Disorders*, **150**, 251–265.

Robin, D.A. and Schienberg, S. (1984). Isolated thalamic lesion and aphasia: A case study. In R.H. Brookshire (Ed.) *Clinical Aphasiology: Conference Proceedings*, pp. 252–261. Minneapolis: BRK.

Robin, D.A. and Schienberg, S. (1990). Subcortical lesions and aphasia. *Journal of Speech and Hearing Disorders*, **55**, 90–100.

Skyhoj-Olsen, T., Bruhn, P. and Oberg, R.G.E. (1986). Cortical hypoperfusion as a possible cause of 'subcortical aphasia'. *Brain*, **109**, 393–410.

Tanridag, O. and Kirshner, H.S. (1987). Language disorders in stroke syndromes of the dominant capsulostriatum: A clinical review. *Aphasiology*, **1**, 107–117.

Tuszynski, M.H. and Petito, C.K. (1988). Ischaemic thalamic aphasia with pathologic confirmation. *Neurology*, **38**, 800–802.

Vallar, G., Papagno, C. and Cappa, S.F. (1988). Latent dysphasia after left hemisphere lesions: A lexical-semantic and verbal memory deficit. *Aphasiology*, **2**, 463–478.

Wallesch, C.W. (1985). Two syndromes of aphasia occurring with ischemic lesions involving the left basal ganglia. *Brain and Language*, **25**, 357–361.

Wallesch, C.W. and Papagno, C. (1988). Subcortical aphasia. In F.C. Rose, R. Whurr and M.A. Wyke (Eds) *Aphasia*, pp. 256–287. London: Whurr Publishers.

Wallesch, C.W., Kornhumber, H.H., Brunner, R.J., Kunz, T., Hollerbach, B. and Suger, G. (1983). Lesions of the basal ganglia, thalamus and deep white matter: Differential effect on language functions. *Brain and Language*, 20, 286–304.

Weinrich, M., Ricaurte, G., Kowall, J., Weinstein, S.C. and Lane, B. (1987). Subcortical aphasia revisited. *Aphasiology*, 1, 119–126.

Wernicke, C. (1874). *Der Aphasische Symptomecomplex*. Breslau: Cohn & Weigert.

Wodarz, R. (1980). Watershed infarctions and computed tomography: A topographical study in cases with stenosis or occlusion of the carotid artery. *Neuroradiology*, 19, 245–248.

Yang, B.J., Yang, T.C., Pan, H.C., Lai, S.J. and Yang, F. (1989). Three variant forms of subcortical aphasia in Chinese stroke patients. *Brain and Language*, 37, 145–162.

# Chapter 8
# Cognitive Neuropsychology and Aphasia: A Critical Analysis

MEREDITH KENNEDY

## Abstract

*In 1973, Marshall and Newcombe were among the first researchers to use the cognitive neuropsychological approach to describe acquired alexia in adults. Since that time a sizeable number of aphasia case studies, which have used the cognitive neuropsychological methodology, have been published. In a number of countries this theoretical approach has become the most prominent approach to aphasiology. Cognitive neuropsychologists have claimed that their methodology enables the researcher to use the results of the detailed language assessment of single cases to inform (a) aphasia theory and (b) models of normal language processing.*

*There has been great debate regarding the soundness of the assumptions associated with cognitive neuropsychological methodology. A number of authors have criticised (a) the use of single case study design, (b) the use of information processing models to model language processes, (c) the modularity assumption, (d) the seriality assumption and, (e) the subtractivity assumption. Other researchers have indicated that there are limitations with the assessment procedures commonly used in the approach. These criticisms do not apply to the cognitive neuropsychological approach alone. However, if the cognitive neuropsychological approach is to deal adequately with aphasia in its complexity, and fulfil its promise to inform models of language processing such criticisms must be explored. One question is to what extent other approaches to aphasia complement or supplant the cognitive neuropsychological approach.*

*This chapter provides an overview of information processing models and their use in the cognitive neuropsychological approach in aphasiology. It discusses the assumptions underlying the approach and evaluates the assessment methods currently used within the cognitive neuropsychological approach. In addition, the need for adaptations to current methodology is discussed.*

# Introduction

Patterns of language impairment in adults who have sustained brain damage have been used to develop models of language processes since the last century. Up until the early 1970s most researchers aimed to develop models of language localisation in the brain using data collected from brain-damaged subjects. More recently researchers have sought to develop models of normal single word processing, unrelated to brain structure, using data from aphasic patients (Morton and Patterson, 1980; Ellis and Young, 1988).

Interest in the cognitive neuropsychological approach in aphasiology was stimulated in 1973 by a paper written by Marshall and Newcombe. These authors were among the first researchers to use the cognitive neuropsychological approach to describe acquired alexia in adults. Since that time a sizeable number of aphasia case studies, which have used the cognitive neuropsychological methodology, have been published. Parisi and Burani (1988) have outlined the four methodological choices of the cognitive neuropsychological approach: (a) use of the single case study design, (b) study of the mind independent of the brain,[1] (c) use of the information processing models of cognitive abilities, and (d) exchange of methods, data and models between cognitive psychology and cognitive neuropsychology. Cognitive neuropsychologists have claimed that their methodology enables the researcher to use the results of the detailed language assessment of single cases to inform both aphasia theory and models of normal language processing. What still remains to be done is an evaluation of the contribution of the cognitive neuropsychological approach to the understanding of aphasic disorders and the development of models of single word processing.

There has been considerable debate regarding the cognitive neuropsychological methodology outlined above. Criticisms of (a) the single case study design (Caplan, 1988; Zurif, Gardner and Brownell, 1989), and (b) the information processing models, in particular the modularity and seriality assumptions and underspecification of the available models (Parisi and Burani, 1988; Schweiger and Brown, 1988; Muller, 1992; Berndt and Mitchum, 1994) are well-known. The assumption that it is possible to consider the mind independent of brain structure, function and evolution has also been criticised to some degree (Schweiger and Brown, 1988; Muller, 1992). Less attention has been given to the fourth aspect of cognitive neuropsychological methodology, that is, the assumption that method, data and models can be exchanged between neuropsychology and cognitive neuropsychology.

---

[1] This feature does not characterise all cognitive neuropsychological approaches. For example, Shallice (1988) took a more moderate view and included discussion of anatomical findings in his review of the contribution of cognitive neuropsychology to the development of models of mental structure.

Many of these criticisms do not apply solely to the cognitive neuropsychological approach. However, these criticisms need to be explored if the cognitive neuropsychological approach is to deal adequately with aphasia in its complexity and fulfil its promise to inform models of single word processing. Indeed, it may be appropriate to consider the extent to which other approaches to the study of aphasia complement or supplant the cognitive neuropsychological approach.

The current chapter has two aims. The first is to evaluate cognitive neuropsychologists' claims that their methodology enables the researcher to use the results of the detailed language assessment of single cases to inform models of normal single word processing. Within cognitive neuropsychology, data from aphasic patients are used to inform both information processing and connectionist models of single word processing. The chapter therefore contains a brief discussion of information processing and connectionist models in aphasiology. The assumption that data collected from patients with aphasia can be used to further develop these models (or indeed any model) of normal function is discussed. In particular the assumptions of fractionation, transparency and subtractivity, which have been made explicit by the approach, are evaluated.

The second aim of the chapter is to evaluate cognitive neuropsychologists' claims that their methodology enables the researcher to use the results of the detailed language assessment of single cases to inform aphasia theory. To achieve this aim the assessment methods currently used to describe the nature of the single word processing deficit in aphasic patients are critically evaluated. The linguistic and non-linguistic abilities that are assessed by the available tests are discussed and assessment procedures which augment currently available cognitive neuropsychological tests are presented.

# Models of single word processing in cognitive neuropsychology

### Information processing models

Research into single word processing has been guided, to a great extent, by models based on the computational metaphor. This metaphor envisions the mind as a computing device and analogises the processes of the mind to the operations of a computer. Early computers were of the information processing (IP) type and the single word processing models based upon them consisted of a number of modules (which contained mental representations) with computational processes that mediated between them. Processing of information occurred in a serial fashion. Although IP models were being used in psychology in the late 1950s and early 1960s it was not until the early 1970s that IP models were influential in cognitive neuropsychology. This is not to say that models were absent from aphasiology prior to the 1970s. Indeed, as Caplan (1987) indicated, the early diagram-makers in aphasiology produced IP-like models.

The recent IP models aim to present the internal structure and function of many types of cognitive processes (memory, attention, language, perception) on the basis of experimental data, collected from normal subjects in cognitive psychology and impaired subjects in cognitive neuropsychology. In the present chapter single word processing models (such as that proposed by Ellis and Young, 1988) are evaluated. These single word processing models, which are predominantly modular with serially organised stages of processing, have been developed from the pattern of co-occurrences and dissociation of symptoms that result from brain damage (Caramazza, 1984). Double dissociation of symptoms, where some patients are impaired in one ability and not in another and other patients show the reverse pattern, have also been used to develop models of single word processing (Saffran, 1982; Riddoch and Humphreys, 1994).

According to Riddoch and Humphreys (1994) double dissociations provide the strongest evidence for identifying processing components within the language system and allow researchers to outline a functional architecture of language processes. This particular approach, however, allows the researcher only to answer the question: How does the system operate in situation A, when compared with its operation in situation B?, not questions such as: How does the system operate in situation A? (Van der Heijen and Stebbins, 1990). Thus, although documentation of double dissociation may be a powerful tool for isolating parallel processes, it is less adequate for identifying serial stages (Sartori, 1988). It follows that the nature of the representations mediating cognitive performance is likely to be under-specified in some models (Berndt and Mitchum, 1994; Riddoch and Humphreys, 1994). Authors such as Caramazza and Hillis (1990) have recognised this limitation and have used descriptions of error types to develop models of single word production.

The modular approach, as it has been presented in single word processing models used by many cognitive neuropsychologists, has been criticised by a number of researchers who have stated that the existence of the proposed modules is antithetical to evolutionary theory (Schweiger and Brown, 1988) and is unjustified biologically (Kosslyn and Intriligator, 1992; Muller, 1992). In fact, there is growing evidence that human neurophysiological functioning is not serial but simultaneously cooperative and parallel (Buckingham, 1986; Schweiger and Brown, 1988). A number of different views exist concerning the use of neuroanatomical information to constrain models of language function.

Hughlings Jackson (1874) indicated that there is not a one-to-one relationship between brain structure and language. More recently, Caramazza (1992) claimed that 'developments in cognitive science concerning the computational structure of cognitive processes can proceed independently of neuroanatomical observations' (p. 85). A more moderate position than the 'against anatomy' position of Hughlings Jackson (1874) and Caramazza (1992) and the 'for anatomy' position of Kosslyn and Intriligator (1992) and Muller (1992) was taken by Stent (1990). He stated that the 'question of whether all psychological phenomena can be explained without residue in terms of neurobiological theories is as yet unresolved. Whereas there is no reason why such reductions should not be possible in principle, the complexity of the nervous system limits the degree to which we can expect to formulate them in practice' (p. 555). In practice then, Caramazza's (1992) directive to proceed independently of neuroanatomical observations in model building may be appropriate for the time being. However, cognitive neuropsychologists obviously would want to consider advances in neurobiological theories in the future.

Criticisms of modularity that are of greater theoretical concern to cognitive neuropsychologists than the biological aspect are the claims that no comprehensive set of principles is used to decide whether any particular function is a module. The only reason for developing a new module appears to be to account for a particular behaviour (Schweiger and Brown, 1988). Thus, as new dissociations are documented modules are allowed to proliferate (Schweiger and Brown, 1988; Tyler, 1992). These criticisms reduce the explanatory adequacy of the single word processing models, making them merely descriptive (Schweiger and Brown, 1988). It is important to note that these criticisms do not apply to all models of cognitive processes that use a modular approach. For example, Fodor (1983) defined the properties of non-modular and modular systems in cognition in terms of a number of variables (for example, speed of processing, automaticity).

Although modular and serially organised models of single word processing have achieved prominence in the last 20 years, neuroscientists are now beginning to adopt another computer metaphor, connectionism, to model cognitive functions. The paradigm shift is not without precedents. For example, models with cascading levels of processing (where each stage of processing can pass on partial information to the next stage without having to wait to complete its computations) (e.g. McClelland, 1979) and bi-directional processing (e.g. Rumelhart, 1975) were proposed in the 1970s. Such models may be viewed as intermediate between models of single word processing commonly found in the neuropsychological literature and connectionist models. Furthermore, many authors who were responsible for developing early models of single word processing (e.g. Shallice and Saffran) are now using the results of the cognitive neuropsychological assessment of aphasic patients to develop connectionist models of language disorders. It would be wrong, therefore, to place models of single word processing and connectionist models in a dichotomous relationship. Whether the move towards connectionist modelling will provide researchers with a more adequate model of single word processing than that provided by IP models is a reasonable question to ask at this point.

## Connectionist models

The study of cognition using connectionist models assumes that processing occurs in a complex network. The network is made up of simple units which are arranged in layers and are joined by connections. Each unit has a level of energy or activation that can spread along its connections. The rate of spread of this activation is controlled by weights on the connections. Complex cognitive processes (such as language) emerge as a consequence of interaction of many simple units (Goschke and Koppelberg, 1990; Harley, 1993). Fundamental to this approach is that the system of representations has the potential to be highly distributed and processed in parallel. This is quite different from the models of single word processing in which information is processed serially. In addition, the emphasis of the connectionist approach on the detailed mechanics of processing is seen to be an advantage over the models of single word processing currently available. Some authors have viewed the obvious parallels between connectionist models and brain structure to be another advantage of connectionism (Kosslyn and Intriligator, 1992).

Connectionist models (which are implemented as computer programs) have been used to model normal language processing predominantly. More recently connectionist models have been used to provide insights into the nature of aphasic language impairments (Martin and Saffran, 1992; Martin, Dell, Saffran and Schwartz, 1994; Schwartz, Dell, Martin and Saffran, 1994). Researchers have 'lesioned' connectionist computer programs (by changing activation levels within the network) in order to simulate aphasic deficits. By examining the types of alterations that need to be made to the connectionist system in order to simulate aphasic deficits, researchers claim that they can describe the underlying cause of the aphasia. It is of interest to note that connectionist models can predict both single and double dissociations without postulating separate processing components (Sartori, 1988). Furthermore, these models are more able to describe degradation of function than the models of single word processing that are currently used within cognitive neuropsychology. The latter concentrate on describing relative sparing and loss of function whereas connectionist models can account for the varying degrees of impairment seen in aphasia (Harley, 1993).

In contrast to these positive accounts of connectionism, both Muller (1992) and Harley (1993) have stated that connectionist networks can sometimes be nearly as difficult to understand as the neural systems that they model. According to Muller (1992), it is possible that connectionist systems may behave as an aphasic would, without their creators knowing exactly why they are behaving in such a way. Thus, aspects of aphasic language may be successfully simulated by a connectionist network but simulation in itself is not explanatory. Stent (1990) pointed out that the human brain or mind may 'belong to a class of phenomena whose very complexity limits the extent to which theories designed to explain them can be successfully reduced by theories developed to explain less complex phenomena' (p. 547). Reductionism of complex language processes to computer programs may not be a realistic or profitable goal.

These reservations aside, it is difficult to predict whether connectionism will make as great an impact in cognitive neuropsychology as the current models of single word processing have done. If there is a paradigm shift away from these models to connectionism in the study of language disorders, it seems reasonable to assume that this change will be similar in effect to that observed when aphasiologists ceased to use the neo-classical model (Goodglass and Kaplan, 1972) in favour of cognitive neuropsychological models (Morton and Patterson, 1980; Ellis and Young, 1988). The change from the neo-classical model to the cognitive neuropsychological models involved swapping one IP model for another. Moving from models of single word processing to connectionism will involve a more significant shift in computer models; from a serial, modular computer model to a model that promotes parallel, distributed processing. Thus, an observable change will occur in the questions that are asked about the nature of aphasia and the way the aphasic disorders are interpreted relative to the connectionist models. Whether there will be subsequent alterations in the research methodology used to collect data on aphasic patients' strengths and weaknesses is still open to question. As yet, no significant changes in assessment procedure used by aphasiologists who have adopted a connectionist approach have occurred. For example, Martin and Saffran (1992) used data collected from an assessment procedure typical of the neuropsychological approach in their connectionist account of deep dysphasia.

## The assumptions of cognitive neuropsychology: fractionation, transparency and subtractivity

One of the goals of cognitive neuropsychology is to propose a model of single word processing as undertaken by the normal brain. Until quite recently these models have been IP models although, as discussed previously, a paradigm shift to connectionist models is currently underway.

Obviously, the most direct way to develop such models of normal language functioning in adults is to study the language of normal adults. In 1984, Caramazza claimed that, as methods for studying the language processes of normal subjects were not available at that time, the study of brain-damaged populations provided the most useful information from which to develop theories of language processing. In using data collected from aphasic patients to develop language processing models, a number of assumptions have to be made concerning the relationship between the normal and damaged systems. Assumptions are made whenever data from aphasic subjects are used to develop models of normal function (see Poeck, 1984, and Kennedy and Murdoch, 1994, for discussion of this point in relation to localisationist models). However, it is the cognitive neuropsychologists who have made their assumptions explicit. There are three main assumptions: the fractionation assumption, the transparency assumption, and the subtractivity assumption.

For over a century aphasiologists have described many patients with a variety of highly specific language disorders following brain damage. These specific language disorders occur in the presence of other intact language abilities and provide unquestionable support for the fractionation assumption (Shallice, 1979). In order for cognitive neuropsychology to work two further assumptions are applied: the transparency assumption and the subtractivity assumption. The transparency assumption states that the observed pathological performance will provide a basis for discerning which component or module of the system is disrupted. The subtractivity assumption states that the performance of the aphasic patient reflects the normal cognitive apparatus *minus* those systems which have been impaired (Saffran, 1982; Caramazza, 1984; Ellis and Young, 1988; Caramazza, 1992). Furthermore, the type of modifications to the system that result from damage must not lead to the creation of new processing structures (Caramazza, 1992).

The transparency and subtractivity assumptions make it possible to build models based on dissociations in the language abilities of aphasic subjects. But it is of these very assumptions that a number of researchers have been critical. Adoption of these assumptions requires that the following findings are ignored:

1.  The move towards parallel processing systems makes subtractivity, which only applies if a modular flow-chart organisation is presupposed, less tenable (Muller, 1992).
2.  The presenting language features may result, not from the effects of a missing or impaired module, but from one of the following mechanisms:
    (a) global reduction in capacity which may selectively impair certain, more vulnerable, aspects of language while leaving others seemingly unaffected (Kilborn, 1991; Blackwell and

Bates, 1994). Most models of single word processing assume a linear relationship between language capacity remaining after brain damage and the observed performance. There may, however, be a non-linear relationship between capacity and performance for some language tasks. For example, receptive agrammatism may not be caused by damage to a module containing 'closed class' items but rather be due to the fact that morphology is particularly vulnerable to a reduction in processing capacity (Blackwell and Bates, 1994).

(b) compensatory mechanisms or strategies employed by the aphasic to deal with the effects of brain damage (Kolk and Heeschen, 1990; Kolk and Hofstede, 1994). Kolk and Heeschen (1990) suggested that language pathology may not be due to direct damage to the language system alone. These authors suggested that aphasic features (for example, agrammatism and paragrammatism) may result from optional strategic choices made by the patient. An example of the optional nature of these adaptation symptoms is provided by Kolk and Hofstede (1994) who showed that a Dutch agrammatic patient was able to alter his spoken output to reduce the proportion of main verbs and subjects omitted under certain task conditions. Kolk and Hofstede (1994) interpreted this finding as indicating that the subject had some degree of control over his sentence production abilities.

(c) failure of brain processes to interact in the same way (Kosslyn and Intriligator, 1992). These authors suggested that damage to one component of the language system may result in alterations to the functioning of the system as a whole. A wide range of neurophysiologic alterations typically occur after focal lesions. These changes in brain function (proximal and distal to the site of lesion) have profound implications for how a given behaviour is ultimately accomplished (Kosslyn and Intriligator, 1992; Gordon, Hart, Lesser and Selnes, 1994). The presenting deficits may therefore be products of the entire changed system, not the misfunctioning of one small component.

Caramazza (1992) defended the cognitive neuropsychologists' position by stating that the problems inherent in the transparency assumption are not specific to this approach but are difficulties which exist in this area of science. Indeed many of the arguments against use of the transparency and subtractivity assumptions in cognitive neuropsychology can be used against any approach (localisationist, connectionist) that uses data collected from brain-damaged patients to develop models of normal function. Although Caramazza (1991, 1992) stated that inferring the structure of normal cognitive processes from impaired performance may not be easy or immediate, it is difficult to ignore these findings against transparency and subtractivity. The only assumption that seems supportable is the fractionation assumption. Saffran's (1982) claim that 'evidence from pathology may be more useful for the purpose (of) isolating cognitive subsystems and describing their general properties than in specifying how particular subsystems are utilised in the normal state' (p. 335) may be very accurate. This statement has also been supported by Shallice (1988) who suggested that cognitive neuropsychological research was more likely to assist in the development of models of normal function by mapping global architecture rather than providing detailed information about the operation of computational models.

Over a decade has passed since Caramazza (1984) stated that there are no methodologies sufficiently powerful to study the workings of the normal brain as it performs complex cognitive functions. It is doubtful whether psycholinguists who routinely use normal subjects to gain insights into the normal language processing system would agree. For example, data collected from *normal* adult subjects using semantic priming tasks (for example, lexical decision and pronunciation tasks) have been used to develop models of visual and spoken word recognition processes. The finding that subjects are faster and more accurate in responding to the second of two semantically/associatively related words (e.g. *bread* and *butter*) than to the second of two unrelated words has been explained by various models (see Neely (1991) for a review of theories of visual word recognition in normal adults). The ultimate goal of the psycholinguistic researchers who use the semantic priming methodology, like the cognitive neuropsychologists, is to develop a complete understanding of the cognitive processes that normal people use in lexical access. It is possible that greater gains may be made through the study of single word processing in normal adults. Using normal adults to develop models of single word processing eliminates the need for the transparency and subtractivity assumptions.

The study of acquired language deficits is essential even if it is not possible to build models from data collected from aphasic subjects. Aphasiologists still have much to learn concerning the patterns of spared and impaired language abilities following brain damage, the reasons for the observed patterns, and appropriate management and rehabilitation strategies. By focusing on describing the range and type of language deficits that occur following brain damage, rather than searching for patients with 'pure syndromes' as is the tendency in cognitive neuropsychology (Shallice, 1988), a more comprehensive account of aphasia will be possible.

The actual tasks which are used by aphasiologists to establish patterns of ability and deficit following brain damage and subsequently to develop hypotheses concerning the nature of the deficit are remarkably similar regardless of the theory by which the results are interpreted. If aphasiologists are to develop theories of aphasia (if not theories of normal processing) a rigorous research methodology is required in order to constrain the choice of alternative theories. As Caramazza (1992) wrote 'we should obtain the kind of detailed experimental observations that do the necessary work in constraining theory' (p. 88). As cognitive neuropsychology is currently the most popular approach to understanding single word processing in aphasic patients, the assessment methods used within this approach should be evaluated in order to determine the extent to which they provide results which are capable of constraining theory.

## Methods of language assessment in aphasiology

Within this section procedures that are currently used to assess the single word processing abilities of aphasic patients are described. The linguistic and non-linguistic abilities that are assessed by the available tests are discussed and experimental methods that will enable the researcher to describe single word processing itself are presented.

In cognitive neuropsychology (and in any approach regardless of the theoretical model chosen), description of aphasic language emphasises the pattern of co-occurrence and dissociation of language symptoms that result from brain damage. The results of language assessments are examined for patterns of symptom dissociation, double dissociation and association, and the types of errors made by the aphasic patient are used to conclude which subsystem (or subsystems) of the normal single word processing model is (are) impaired. In 1992, an assessment of single word processing based on the cognitive neuropsychological approach, Psycholinguistic Assessment of Language Processing (PALPA) (Kay, Lesser and Coltheart, 1992), was published. Many of the tests of the PALPA were adapted from assessments used by researchers in published case studies.

Cognitive neuropsychological assessments of the single word processing system of aphasic patients consist of assessments such as word to picture matching (spoken and written), picture naming (spoken and written), repetition, discrimination of minimal pairs, and word/nonword decision tasks. Variables such as word imageability, word frequency, word length and grammatical class are manipulated within the subtests. It is assumed that the tests included in this assessment (and those experiments on which they are based) can be used to (a) interrogate the functioning of selected components of a patient's single word processing system, and (b) infer which components are intact and which are impaired from the pattern of performance shown by the patient (Ellis, Franklin and Crerar, 1994).

Two arguments have been used against language assessments such as the PALPA as well as analyses of connected language which are often collected to supplement standard language tests in the description of the language of aphasic patients. First, it is well-recognised that such assessments are only indirect assessment methods of the internal workings of the single word processor of aphasic adults (Parisi, 1985; Bradley, 1989). Both Parisi (1985) and Crain (1987) indicated that most language assessments (such as the PALPA) test many non-linguistic abilities in addition to language processing abilities of the patient. The non-linguistic abilities that are needed to perform on a language assessment include motor skills, working memory, attention and perception abilities and motivation. Second, it is assumed that linguistic variables are relevant in the description of the language of aphasic patients. Indeed, the authors of currently used aphasia tests, such as the PALPA, have manipulated linguistic variables in their assessments (e.g. word class, length, imageability, frequency) even though there is no evidence to suggest that these variables are theoretically important in aphasia. This is not to say that the language deficits of English aphasic patients do not vary along these dimensions. Of importance is the concept that a description of the linguistic variables of aphasic patients' language is just that, a description and therefore is not explanatory. This point is often overlooked by many aphasiologists. For example, it has been indicated by some aphasiologists that the presence of difficulty producing morphology in an aphasic patient means that there is a deficit in the patient's morphological system. The Competition Model (MacWhinney and Bates, 1989), for example, provides an alternative account of deficits demonstrated by aphasic patients in language assessments to those characterisations provided by cognitive neuropsychologists.

Briefly, the Competition Model was developed from the results of the cross-linguistic study of normal adults and children and has been used to interpret the results of sentence comprehension assessments and samples of spontaneous speech in aphasic adults. The Competition Model provides predictions about language performance in a given situation (for example, following brain damage or when degraded auditory stimuli are used with unimpaired adults) based on two quantifiable principles: (a) cue validity and (b) cue cost. Cue validity refers to the information value of a given phonological, lexical, and morphological or syntactic form within a particular language. Cue cost refers to the type and amount of processing associated with activation and deployment of a given linguistic form, when cue validity is held constant. The amount of processing required is influenced by variables such as the perceivability of the linguistic form, ease of articulation and demands on memory. Thus, linguistic forms with high cue validity and low cue cost are predicted to be more resistant to impairment in aphasia than linguistic forms with low cue validity and high cue cost. For example, in aphasia pragmatics and syntax are more resistant to impairment than grammatical morphology (Bates and Wulfeck, 1989). The former can be considered to have high cue validity and low cue cost whereas the latter is a linguistic form of low cue validity and high cue cost. From the results of their studies Bates, Wulfeck and MacWhinney (1991) concluded that aphasia results from deficits in the processes by which linguistic knowledge is accessed and deployed. Classes of linguistic information that are high in cue cost are selectively impaired by this processing limitation relative to classes that are low in cue cost. Thus, the influence of non-linguistic factors on an aphasic's performance in language assessment is taken into account and an alternative reason for the presence of morphological deficits in an aphasic patient is provided by the Competition Model. A shortcoming of the Competition Model is that the processing limitation that aphasic patients are deemed to have is not well specified and is suggested to be related to factors as diverse as attention, the perceivability of the linguistic form, the ease of articulation of a linguistic form and demands on memory.

There are two general factors (at least) that may affect processing. These are (a) non-linguistic abilities such those involved in decision-making, memory, motor skills and picture recognition, and (b) language specific access and retrieval processes (which may or may not be common to all aspects of language). As aphasiologists are predominantly interested in determining the nature of the language disorder of the aphasic patient, it is essential that researchers can say with a reasonable degree of confidence that the non-linguistic deficits of the patient are not significantly affecting the assessment results. It is obvious that researchers cannot ensure that an aphasic patient will not have non-linguistic impairments that will affect his/her performance on language tasks. A good research methodology will ensure that for all tasks the demands on memory and decision-making are kept reasonably constant for all tasks while the language processing task is manipulated (Stewart and Kennedy, 1995).

The other important variable when examining language functions is the patient's ability to perform in tasks of varying linguistic processing load (where all factors are kept constant except the degree of processing required). To my knowledge there is no model available in aphasiology that outlines the language processing system and its operation across a range of processing tasks. In 1988, Stark used Karmiloff-Smith's (1986) developmental model of the language processing system to discuss the effect of linguistic processing load on aphasic performance. The model claims that the language processing system contains linguistic representations and the procedures that operate directly upon them. In addition, it includes the mechanisms that enable the speaker to consciously access linguistic information in a variety of language tasks. Karmiloff-Smith (1986) proposed four levels of representation in the language processing system. These levels, from lowest to highest developmental level of processing with examples of assessments which tap each level, are as follows: (i) implicit knowledge – linguistic representations which cannot be operated upon separately (no assessment procedures available), (ii) primary explication – the process by which the representations can be accessed internally (real-time lexical decision tasks), (iii) secondary explication – the process by which the representations can be accessed consciously (word–picture matching), and (iv) tertiary explication – where links or commonalities across codes can be drawn (semantic similarity judgements).

In order to more fully understand the nature of aphasic disorders, experimental procedures should enable the researcher to determine the level of processing at which the aphasic patient is having difficulty. No methodology available at this time allows researchers to assess unambiguously the underlying linguistic representations without some processing occurring. The status of the representation is currently inferred from aphasic patients' performance in language tasks (Bates, Wulfeck and MacWhinney, 1991; McEntee and Kennedy, 1995; Milberg and Blumstein, 1981).[2] What researchers are able to directly investigate to gain a greater knowledge of the nature of aphasia is the aphasic patient's ability to perform in a number of language tasks such as real-time lexical processing tasks, tasks that involve conscious access of linguistic representations (e.g. word–picture matching, semantic similarity judgements) and naturalistic language tasks.

In general cognitive neuropsychologists have not considered that an aphasic patient's abilities to process language in real-time may differ from his/her ability to perform in tasks that involve conscious access of linguistic representations. Cognitive neuropsychologists have used language tasks that require conscious access of the linguistic representations in their assessment of aphasic patients. In contrast, experimental methodologies which attempt to measure subjects' ability to process information in real-time with a minimal conscious component have been developed by psycholinguists.

The distinction between automatic/real-time processes and conscious processes involved in lexical access is a central issue in contemporary cognitive neuroscience. The fact that some researchers have used semantic priming methodologies to develop models of cognitive processes in normal people has been mentioned in this chapter. These models of single word processing differ from cognitive neuropsychological models. An example of one model of lexical processing is that of Fodor (1983). Fodor (1983) suggested that the cognitive system consists of two qualitatively different types of components: (a) perceptual-input systems, and (b) central systems. The perceptual-input systems are responsible for

---

[2] Many authors have indicated that the underlying representation is intact in aphasic patients and have suggested that the deficit is in the access and/or retrieval of the representation (Milberg and Blumstein, 1981; Caplan and Hildebrant, 1986; Milberg, Blumstein and Dworetzky, 1987, 1988; Chenery, Ingram and Murdoch, 1990; Bates, Wulfeck and McWhinney, 1991; Tyler, 1992; McEntee and Kennedy, 1995).

input analysis and are modular, domain specific and mandatory, and work in a data driven bottom-up fashion on in-coming information. The central systems are modular and integrate different types of perceptual information.[3] At first glance, Fodor's model may be mistaken for the skeleton of the single word processing model of Ellis and Young (1988). That is, the non-modular semantic system receives input from the incoming data driven input analysis and input lexicon modules. The important difference between the two models is that Fodor distinguishes between the automatic and unconscious processing performed by the input-perceptual systems in real-time tasks and the conscious processing performed by the central systems in problem solving and decision-making tasks. The model of Ellis and Young (1988) does not.

The methodology used to assess real-time access to linguistic structures (for example, lexical decision tasks) has been adopted by aphasiologists to explore the lexical processing abilities (visual and auditory) of aphasic patients (e.g. Milberg and Blumstein, 1981; Blumstein, Milberg and Shrier, 1982; Milberg, Blumstein and Dworetzky, 1987, 1988). These authors have adopted Posner and Snyder's (1975) suggestion that two types of processes interact during normal lexical access. The two types of processes are: (a) automatic processes that are effortless, fast acting, of short duration, and not under voluntary control and (b) controlled processes that are slower acting, under a subject's control, and are influenced by a subject's expectancies or attentional demands.

The evidence collected from lexical decision tasks suggests that the single word processing abilities of some aphasic patients seem to be better preserved on tests of automatic processing (that is, on-line assessments) than would be expected from their performance on standard aphasia tests (that is, off-line assessments) (Milberg and Blumstein, 1981; Blumstein et al., 1982; Milberg et al., 1987, 1988). Similar findings have been reported in on-line assessments of syntactic processing Tyler, 1988, 1992). Such findings led Flores d'Arcais (1988) to propose that the language deficits in the various forms of aphasia may not be to do with the processing of language itself as processing can occur automatically and successfully under certain conditions (on-line tasks). It has been suggested that deficits demonstrated by aphasic patients are due to difficulties that the aphasic patient has in consciously or intentionally using his/her preserved language processing abilities (Flores d'Arcais, 1988; Tyler, 1988, 1992). Thus, a dissociation, which is not easily accounted for by current single word processing models used within cognitive neuropsychology, is presented. According to Schacter, McAndrews and Moscovitch (1988) the role of conscious processes in aphasic disorders will have to be taken into account by models of single word processing.

---

[3] In addition to the two systems proposed by Fodor (1983), Friederici (1990) suggested the existence of a third type of system, the interface system. The interface system supposedly represents the declarative knowledge that underlies the procedural perceptual-input systems.

Two assumptions have been made by those researchers who have used assessments of automatic processing with aphasic patients. They are: (a) that there are two types of processes that operate during normal lexical access and that it is possible to assess each process independently of the other, and (b) that lexical decision tasks assess the integrity of the semantic system. Whether these assumptions are valid is an important point to consider. Firstly, in relation to point (a), the idea that there are two distinct processes involved in lexical processing (Ponser and Snyder, 1975) is not supported by a number of researchers who use priming methodology in the study of visual word recognition. For example, some authors have suggested that controlled processing alone can account for priming (Becker, 1980) whereas others have suggested that it is unlikely that only two mechanisms can explain the complexity of semantic priming effects that have been documented (Neely, 1991). Although *auditory* priming is used with aphasic patients (rather than visual priming described by Neely, 1991[4]), the occurrence of semantic priming in aphasic patients may not necessarily suggest that automatic lexical access procedures are intact. However, the results of the experiments of Milberg and Blumstein can be interpreted as indicating that some aphasic patients are able to undertake *some degree* of lexical processing. Furthermore, in relation to point (b), Moss and Marslen-Wilson (1993) showed recently that semantic priming methodology using associated primes such as *dog–cat* assesses a different process from priming methodologies that use semantically related primes such as *banana–curved*. It was suggested that associative priming does not necessarily reflect access to lexical semantic representations. Research on the semantic priming abilities of aphasic patients has typically used associative primes (Blumstein et al., 1982; Milberg et al., 1988) and therefore may not provide adequate information concerning the ability of the subjects to access lexical semantic representations.

Whether the semantic structure needed to support semantic priming effects is equivalent to that required to support accurate performance in semantic decision tasks has been queried also (Caramazza, Hillis, Rapp and Romani, 1990). In order to discuss Caramazza et al.'s (1990) comment it is necessary to look to research that compares the performance of aphasic patients on lexical decision tasks and off-line tasks that use the same test materials (Chenery, Ingram and Murdoch, 1990; Tyler, 1992). In these experiments only one independent variable exists, that is, the degree of conscious processing required to perform each task. These researchers, like others who have compared aphasic patients' performance on real-time lexical decision tasks and standard language assessments (Blumstein et al., 1982; Tyler, 1988), have found that they

---

[4] It is important to note that some authors have presented visual and auditory input as parallel processes within their models of lexical access (see, for example, the work of Forster, 1976; and Caron, 1992).

perform better on lexical decision tasks than off-line tasks. It is suggested that Caramazza et al.'s (1990) criticism is not supported by the available evidence.

It is possible to conclude from the discussion thus far that the assessment of the language abilities of aphasic patients should consider (a) the aspect of language being assessed, (b) the processing load of the task,[5] and (c) the decision-making and other non-linguistic demands of the tasks. Although it has been stated previously in this chapter that aphasic data should not be used to develop models of normal function, the use of models of normal function to guide assessment of aphasic data is not precluded. After all, aphasic language is formulated by a once normal language system following modification. Therefore, it is logical to suggest that models of normal language can be used as a starting point for the assessment of aphasic patients. Psycholinguistic research of normal subjects has utilised linguistic levels of description (semantics, syntax, pragmatics and phonology). As long as these levels are assumed to be descriptive and not explanatory and interaction between levels of language is considered, the use of these linguistic levels in aphasiology seems reasonable.

An assessment approach is needed in which the researcher varies the processing load of the tasks if insight is to be gained into the nature of aphasic deficits and areas of preserved ability are to be documented. Obviously, the tasks chosen should be carefully selected in that the researcher should ensure that the experiment is tapping the required language level and that the experiment should involve variation of the language processing requirements of the task only. The motor, memory and decision-making load should be kept constant across tasks. Whether the processing limitation is specific to one level of language is also an interesting issue. In order to make these points more explicit, I will provide an example of work in progress (Stewart, in preparation; Stewart and Kennedy, 1995).

We have developed directly comparable on-line and off-line semantic processing assessments and have attempted to keep meta-linguistic and non-linguistic aspects of all the tasks constant. The semantic priming task compares facilitation from semantically related primes with unrelated primes. The effect of differing semantic relationships will be explored. The off-line semantic task uses the same auditory stimuli in conscious judgement tasks and is similar to the synonym judgement tasks found in the PALPA. The demands on memory and decision-making are equivalent in the two tasks. The results of the on-line and off-

---

[5] I prefer to use the term 'processing load' rather than make the dichotomous automatic-controlled distinction because of the lack of certainty regarding the processing mechanism that is utilised in lexical decision tasks. Based on Stark's (1988) application of Karmiloff-Smith's (1986) model, lexical decision tasks have a low processing load whereas semantic similarity judgements have a high processing load.

line assessments will be compared in order to determine if there is any difference in performance between tasks of differing linguistic processing load. We also wish to determine if the pattern of performance is similar in other language domains. In this instance, we selected phonology. The equivalent on-line phonological task compares facilitation from a phonologically related prime with unrelated primes (we are still doing pilot work to decide on the most appropriate phonological relationship). The equivalent off-line phonological task is similar to phonological-relatedness judgement tasks found in the PALPA. The patient's performance across language domains will be compared and similarities or differences in performances in semantic tasks and phonological tasks will be documented. At this point differences in performance related to unequal data set sizes in the possible number of semantic relationships and the possible number of phonological relationships will have to be taken into account. It is hoped that these comparisons will provide insight into the degree of specificity of the language processing deficit of the patient.

The purpose of the experiments is to describe the on-line and off-line semantic processing abilities of a group of aphasic patients and to determine the degree of specificity of any language processing impairment. The data that are collected will be examined for commonalities across patients and individual variations will also be considered. As in cognitive neuropsychology, the best method for undertaking this detailed description of aphasia is a series of single-patient case studies (Caramazza, 1984; Caramazza and Badecker, 1989). This methodology allows for an exhaustive analysis of the language abilities of the individual patient (Caramazza, 1984) but also reduces the risk of idiosyncratic results being used to constrain aphasia theory. The researcher can evaluate the variability of performance across aphasic patients and is provided with an opportunity to look for replication of findings.

It is not suggested that the on-line and off-line assessment tasks will replace a detailed psycholinguistic profile. We merely propose that such assessment procedures will be an addition to the test procedures available to the researcher. That is, language assessments such as the PALPA could be used to describe the type of language problem that the patient has in language tasks (for example, whether the patient has problems that could be described as semantic or/and phonological). Matched on-line and off-line assessments that control non-linguistic variables and vary linguistic processing load should provide the researcher with a greater insight into the patient's single word processing abilities.

In essence, the suggestion is similar to Crystal's (1988) argument that a detailed description of the aphasic patient's language abilities and impairments is required if researchers are to gain greater insight into the nature of aphasia. Following Crystal's suggestion, the description is based on linguistic levels (that is, semantics, phonology). The difference is that the suggested approach is experimental rather than based on the analysis of connected speech. The advantages of the experimental approach are that the linguistic level to be assessed can be looked at in isolation, that non-linguistic and meta-linguistic variables can be controlled and the linguistic processing load of the task can be manipulated. Exactly what the relationship is among lexical decision tasks, language tasks involving a greater amount of linguistic processing, and natural language use in conversation has not been discussed in any detail by researchers from either a cognitive neuropsychological or psycholinguistic background. It is understandable that researchers use experiments, which can be tightly controlled, to isolate the nature of the aphasic impairment. At some point though, the aphasic patient's performance in a natural language situation must be evaluated.

## Conclusions

Cognitive neuropsychologists use data from aphasic patients to develop and constrain single word processing models, which are modular and serially organised. Double dissociations are viewed as the most robust method for outlining the functional architecture for a given task (Riddoch and Humphreys, 1994). Although double dissociations of aphasic symptoms can delineate language activities that occur in parallel in a given patient, it is questionable whether double dissociations on cognitive neuropsychological assessments alone can provide sufficient data to develop (a) hypotheses concerning the nature of the language impairment of the patient, and (b) detailed models of single word processing in normal adults.

Connectionism is a more recent approach to modelling aphasic deficits and normal single word processes. Although connectionism is not without limitations, it is interesting to note that researchers who use this model aim to understand aphasic disorders more fully rather than use the disorders to develop models of normal single word processing (see, for example, the Competition Model, MacWhinney and Bates, 1989). Given the many reservations concerning the use of data from aphasic patients to develop models of normal single word processing, this seems a sensible use of a model. Greater insight into normal language processing may be gained through the study of language processes in normal adults.

It seems best to consider that most language tasks test the *language processor* of the aphasic patient rather than the functioning of modules of the normal single word processing system. If researchers are to come anywhere near understanding the nature of aphasia carefully controlled and matched assessments which vary language processing load should be used in order to gain a comprehensive description of the language strengths and weaknesses of aphasic patients. The assessment results could then be used to further specify the nature of the disorder in aphasia. That is, it may be possible for researchers to be more specific about the nature of the processing deficit that exists in aphasia. The points raised in this chapter add to the growing awareness in aphasiology that knowledge about the nature of acquired language disorders will only be gained if researchers use valid, reliable and well-controlled experiments (Caramazza, 1992; Odell, Hashi, Miller and McNeil, 1995).

## Acknowledgements

The author wishes to thank Fiona Stewart, Nick Miller and Irmgarde Horsley for their valuable comments on earlier drafts of this chapter.

## References

Bates, E. and Wulfeck, B. (1989). Comparative aphasiology: a cross-linguistic approach to language breakdown. *Aphasiology*, 3, 111–142.

Bates, E., Wulfeck, B. and MacWhinney, B. (1991). Cross-linguistic research in aphasia: An overview. *Brain and Language*, 41, 123–148.

Becker, C.A. (1980). Semantic context effects in visual word recognition: An analysis of semantic strategies. *Memory and Cognition*, 8, 493–512.

Berndt, R. S. and Mitchum, C. C. (1994). Approaches to the rehabilitation of 'phonological assembly': Elaborating the model of nonlexical reading. In M.J. Riddoch and G.W. Humphreys (Eds) *Cognitive Neuropsychology and Cognitive Rehabilitation*, pp. 503–526. Hove, UK: Lawrence Erlbaum.

Blackwell, A. and Bates, E. (1994). Inducing agrammatic profiles in normals. *Proceedings of the Sixteenth Annual Conference of the Cognitive Science Society*. August 13–16, Atlanta, Georgia.

Blumstein, S.E., Milberg, W. and Shrier, R. (1982). Semantic processing in aphasia: Evidence from an auditory lexical decision task. *Brain and Language*, 17, 301–315.

Bradley, D. (1989). Cognitive science and the language/cognition distinction. *Aphasiology*, 3, 755–757.

Buckingham, H. W. (1986). Language, the mind and psychophysical parallelism. In I. Gopnik and M. Gopnik (Eds), *From Models to Modules*. Norwood, New Jersey: Albex Publishers.

Caplan, D. (1987). *Neurolinguistics and Linguistic Aphasiology*. Cambridge: Cambridge University Press.

Caplan, D. (1988). On the role of group studies in neuropsychological and pathopsychological research. *Cognitive Neuropsychology*, 5, 535–548.

Caplan, D. and Hildebrant, N. (1986). Language deficits and the theory of syntax: A reply to Grodzinsky. *Brain and Language*, 27, 168–177.

Caramazza, A. (1984). The logic of neuropsychological research and the problem of patient classification in aphasia. *Brain and Language*, 21, 9–20.

Caramazza, A. (1991). Data, statistics, and theory: A comment on Bates, McDonald, MacWhinney, and Applebaums's 'A maximal likelihood procedure for the analysis of group and individual data in aphasia research'. *Brain and Language*, 41, 43–51.

Caramazza, A. (1992). Is cognitive neuropsychology possible? *Journal of Cognitive Neuroscience* 4, 80–95.

Caramazza, A. and Badecker, W. (1989). Patient classification in neuropsychological research. *Brain and Cognition*, 10, 256–295.

Caramazza, A. and Hillis, A. E. (1990). Where do semantic errors come from? *Cortex*, 26, 95–122.

Caramazza, A., Hillis, A.E., Rapp, B.C. and Romani, C. (1990). The multiple semantics hypothesis: Multiple confusions? *Cognitive Neuropsychology*, 7, 161–189.

Caron, J. (1992). *An Introduction to Psycholinguistics*. New York: Harvester Wheatsheaf.

Chenery, H. J., Ingram, J. C. L. and Murdoch, B. E. (1990). Automatic and volitional processing in aphasia. *Brain and Language*, 38, 215–232.

Crain, S. (1987). On performability: structure and process in language understanding. *Clinical Linguistics and Phonetics*, 1, 127–145.

Crystal, D. (1988). Linguistic levels in aphasia. In F. Rose, R. Whurr and M. Wyke (Eds) *Aphasia*. London: Whurr Publishers.

Ellis, A.W. and Young, A. (1988). *Human Cognitive Neuropsychology*. London: Lawrence Erlbaum.

Ellis, A., Franklin, S. and Crerar, A. (1994). Cognitive neuropsychology and the remediation of disorders of spoken language. In M.J. Riddoch and G.W. Humphreys (Eds) *Cognitive Neuropsychology and Cognitive Rehabilitation*, pp. 287–317. Hove, UK: Lawrence Erlbaum.

Flores d' Arcais, G.B. (1988). Automatic processes in language comprehension. In G. Denes (Ed.) *Perspectives on Cognitive Neuropsychology*, pp. 91–114. Hillsdale: Lawrence Erlbaum.

Fodor, J.A. (1983). *The Modularity of Mind*. Cambridge, MA: MIT.

Forster, K.I. (1976). Accessing the mental lexicon. In R.J. Wales and E. Walker (Eds) *New Approaches to Language Mechanisms*, pp. 257–287. Amsterdam: North-Holland.

Friederici, A.D. (1990). On the properties of cognitive modules. *Psychology Research*, 52, 175–180.

Goodglass, H. and Kaplan, E. (1972). *The Assessment of Aphasia and Related Disorders*. Philadelphia: Lea & Febiger.

Gordon, B., Hart, J., Lesser, R.P. and Selnes, O.A. (1994). Recovery and its implications for cognitive neuroscience. *Academy of Aphasia Conference Proceedings*.

Goschke, T. and Koppelberg, D. (1990). Connectionist representation, semantic compositionality and the instability of concept structure. *Psychology Research*, 52, 253–270.

Harley, T. A. (1993). Connectionist approaches to language disorders. *Aphasiology*, 7, 221–249.

Jackson, H. (1874). On the nature of the duality of the brain. *Medical Press and Circular*, 1, 19, 41, 63.

Karmiloff-Smith, A. (1986). From meta-processes to conscious access: evidence from children's metalinguistic and repair data. *Cognition*, 23, 95–147.

Kay, J., Lesser, R. and Coltheart, M. (1992). *Psycholinguistic Assessment of Language Processing in Aphasia*. Hove, UK: Lawrence Erlbaum.

Kennedy, M. and Murdoch, B.E. (1994). Thalamic aphasia and striato-capsular aphasia as independent aphasic syndromes: a review. *Aphasiology*, 8, 303–313.

Kilborn, K. (1991). Selective impairment of grammatical morphology due to induced stress in normal listeners: Implications for aphasia. *Brain and Language*, 41, 275–288.

Kolk, H. and Heeschen, C. (1990). Adaptation symptoms and impairment symptoms in Broca's aphasia. *Aphasiology*, 4, 221–232.

Kolk, H. and Hofstede, B. (1994). The choice of ellipsis: A case study of stylistic shifts in an agrammatic speaker. *Brain and Language*, 47, 507–509.

Kosslyn, S.M. and Intriligator, J.M. (1992). Is cognitive neuropsychology plausible? The perils of sitting on a one-legged stool. *Journal of Cognitive Neuroscience*, 4, 96–106.

Marshall, J. and Newcombe, F. (1973). Patterns of paralexia: A psycholinguistic approach. *Journal of Psycholinguistic Research*, 2, 175–199.

Martin, N. and Saffran, E.M. (1992). A computational account of deep dysphasia: Evidence from a single case study. *Brain and Language*, 43, 240–274.

Martin, N., Dell, G.S., Saffran, E.M. and Schwartz, M.F. (1994). Origins of paraphasias in deep dyslexia: Testing the consequences of a decay impairment to an interactive spreading activation model of lexical retrieval. *Brain and Language*, 47, 609–660.

McClelland, J.L. (1979). On time-relations of mental processes: an examination of systems of processes in cascade. *Psychological Review*, 86, 287–330.

McEntee, L. J. and Kennedy, M. (1995). Profiling agrammatic spoken language: towards a Government and Binding Framework. *European Journal of Disorders of Communication*, 30, 317–332.

MacWhinney, B. and Bates, E. (1989). *The Crosslinguistic Study of Sentence Processing*. New York: Cambridge University Press.

Milberg, W. and Blumstein, S.E. (1981). Lexical decision in aphasia: Evidence for semantic processing. *Brain and Language*, 14, 371–385.

Milberg, W., Blumstein, S.E. and Dworetzky, B. (1987). Processing of lexical ambiguities in aphasia. *Brain and Language*, 31, 138–150.

Milberg, W., Blumstein, S.E. and Dworetzky, B. (1988). Phonological processing and lexical access in aphasia. *Brain and Language*, 34, 279–293.

Morton, J. and Patterson, K.E. (1980). A new attempt at an interpretation, or an attempt at a new interpretation. In M. Coltheart, K. Patterson and J.C. Marshall (Eds) *Deep Dyslexia*. London: Routledge & Kegan Paul.

Moss, H.E. and Marslen-Wilson, W.D. (1993). Access to word meanings during spoken language comprehension: effects of sentential semantic context. *Journal of Experimental Psychology*, 19, 1254–1276.

Muller, R-A. (1992). Modularism, holism, connectionism: old conflicts and new perspectives on aphasiology and neuropsychology. *Aphasiology*, 6, 443–475.

Neely, J.H. (1991). Semantic priming effects in visual word recognition: A selected review of current findings and theories. In D. Besner and G.W. Humphreys (Eds) *Basic Processes in Reading: Visual Word Recognition*. London: Lawrence Erlbaum.

Odell, K.H., Hashi, M., Miller, S.B. and McNeil, M.R. (1995). A critical look at the notion of selective impairment. *Clinical Aphasiology*, 23, 1–8.

Parisi, D. (1985). A procedural approach to the study of aphasia. *Brain and Language*, 26, 1–15.

Parisi, D. and Burani, C. (1988). Observations on theoretical models in neuropsychology of language. In G. Denes, C. Semenza and P. Bisiacchi (Eds) *Perspectives on Cognitive Neuropsychology*. London: Lawrence Erlbaum.

Poeck, K. (1984). What do we mean by 'aphasic syndromes'? A neurologist's view. *Brain and Language*, 20, 79–89.

Posner, M.I. and Snyder, C.R.R. (1975). Attention and cognitive control. In R.L. Solso (Ed.) *Information Processing and Cognition: The Loyola Symposium*. Hillsdale: Lawrence Erlbaum.

Riddoch, M.J. and Humphreys, G.W. (1994). Cognitive neuropsychology and cognitive rehabilitation: A marriage of equal partners? In M.J. Riddoch and G.W. Humphreys (Eds) *Cognitive Neuropsychology and Cognitive Rehabilitation*, pp. 1–15. Hove, UK: Lawrence Erlbaum.

Rumelhart, D.E. (1975). Notes on a schema for stories. In D.G. Bobrow and A.M. Collins (Eds) *Representation and Understanding*, pp. 211–236. New York: Academic Press.

Saffran, E.M. (1982). Neuropsychological approaches to the study of language. *British Journal of Psychology*, 73, 317–337.

Sartori, G. (1988). From neuropsychological data to theory and vice-versa. In G. Denes, P. Bisiacchi, C. Semenza and E. Andrewsky (Eds) *Perspectives in Cognitive Neuropsychology*, pp. 59–73. London: Lawrence Erlbaum.

Schacter, D.L., McAndrews, M.P. and Moscovitch, M. (1988). Access to consciousness: Dissociations between implicit and explicit knowledge in neuropsychological syndromes. In L. Weiskrantz (Ed.) *Thought Without Language*, pp. 242–278. Oxford: Oxford University Press.

Schwartz, M.F., Dell, G.S., Martin, N. and Saffran, E.M. (1994). Normal and aphasic naming in an interactive spreading activation model. *Brain and Language*, 47,. 391–394.

Schweiger, A. and Brown, J. (1988). Minds, models and modules. *Aphasiology*, 2, 531–543.

Shallice, T. (1979). Case study approach in neuropsychological research. *Journal of Clinical Neuropsychology*, 1, 183–211.

Shallice, T. (1988). *From Neuropsychology to Mental Structure*. Cambridge: Cambridge University Press.

Stark, J.A. (1988). Aspects of automatic versus controlled processing, monitoring, metalinguistic tasks and related phenomena in aphasia. In W. Dressler (Ed.) *Linguistic Analyses of Aphasic Language*. New York: Springer Verlag.

Stent, G.S. (1990). The poverty of neurophilosophy. *Journal of Medicine and Philosophy*, 15, 539–557.

Stewart, F. (in preparation). *Automatic and Controlled Language Processing in Healthy Elderly and Aphasic Subjects*. Doctoral dissertation, University of Newcastle-upon-Tyne.

Stewart, F. and Kennedy, M. (1995) *A comparison of automatic and intentional language processing in healthy elderly and aphasic subjects*. Paper presented at the British Aphasiology Society conference, University of York.

Tyler, L.K. (1988). Spoken language comprehension in a fluent aphasic patient. *Cognitive Neuropsychology*, 5, 375–400.

Tyler, L.K. (1992). *Spoken Language Comprehension: An Experimental Approach to Disordered and Normal Processing*. Cambridge, Mass.: MIT Press.

Van der Heijen, A.H.C. and Stebbins, S. (1990). The information-processing approach. *Psychology Research*, 52, 197–206.

Warrington, E.K. and Shallice, T. (1984). Category specific semantic impairments. *Brain*, 107, 829–853.

Zurif, E.B., Gardner, H. and Brownell, H.H. (1989). The case against the case against group studies. *Brain and Cognition*, 10, 237–255.

# Chapter 9
# Limitations of Models of Sentence Production: Evidence from Cantonese Data of Normal and Aphasic Speakers

EDWIN M.-L. YIU AND LINDA WORRALL

## Abstract

*Most studies of both normal and abnormal language processing have been conducted in primarily European languages. Languages with different linguistic structures would provide opportunities to investigate the universality of language processing. There are several features of Cantonese grammatical structure which make it an interesting language to test. This chapter discusses research which suggests an increased use of elliptical sentences by Cantonese aphasia subjects. Elliptical sentences are more acceptable in normal Cantonese narratives and these results suggest that Cantonese speaking people with aphasia opt to use more elliptical sentences and therefore compensate for their impairment. Compensation is an issue that must be addressed further in models of normal and impaired sentence processing.*

## Introduction

The differences between using normal and impaired subjects to study language processing lie in the dissimilarity of the neuronal pathways, the behaviour of the subject and the different environmental context of an impaired person and a normal person. A major difference is the ability of the impaired individual to compensate. Using the World Health Organization's framework of impairment, disability and handicap (WHO, 1980), compensation occurs at the impairment level (i.e. the brain compensates for lost function), at the disability level (the individual develops strategies to compensate in everyday life) and at the handicap level (the individual and society compensate in terms of their expectations).

184

This chapter focuses on the compensation issue and discusses how this limits the usefulness of models of normal language processing. It does not suggest that models based on normal subjects cannot be used to predict phenomena observed in impaired individuals such as people with aphasia, nor does it suggest that data from impaired individuals cannot be used to inform models or theories of normal language processing. It does, however, draw attention to the issue of compensation and suggests that this cannot be ignored when interpreting data from impaired or normal subjects.

There is general consensus amongst neurobiological researchers that there is a high degree of plasticity of neural networks and that networks are 'rewired' and 'reprogrammed', as a result of a lesion (Flohr, 1988). Indeed, many therapeutic approaches to aphasia are based upon potential post-lesion plasticity and could be termed re-establishment or reorganisational strategies (Seron, 1984). Hence, there is compensation by the brain to the lesion.

There is not only compensation at the neurobiological level but also at the behavioural level. One theory which attempts to describe why aphasic patients exhibit agrammatic speech is the compensation or adaptation hypothesis (Kolk and van Grunsven, 1985; Kolk and Heeschen, 1990). This hypothesis suggests that the reduced sentence length, with the use of primarily content words in agrammatic speech, is a deliberate attempt by the patient to compensate for their difficulty in forming longer complex structures. Reduced sentence length can also be achieved by using elliptical sentences in some languages (e.g. Chinese, see Packard, 1990). If agrammatic speakers of these languages are making compensations, it is reasonable to expect them to produce a large proportion of elliptical sentences so as to reduce the sentence length. Since English discourse does not offer much opportunity for the production of elliptical sentences, evidence from other languages will help to test the hypothesis. A study will therefore be reported here to show how elliptical sentences are produced extensively by Cantonese agrammatic speakers.

Cantonese is a Chinese dialect which, like English, has as its primary word order, subject (S) – verb (V) – object (O). It is, however, a topic prominent language, which means a sentence takes a topic–comment structure in contrast to the subject–complement structure in English (Tsao, 1990; Li and Thompson, 1981). In Cantonese discourse, the topic of a sentence can be omitted if it is understood or has been mentioned previously in the sentence chain, thus leaving the sentence elliptical (Tsao, 1990). Therefore, elliptical sentences are frequently produced in Cantonese connected speech.

The process that a speaker uses to translate a message into a string of words entails not only the selection of appropriate words, but also the correct ordering of these words. The production of morphological structures (e.g. verb inflections, plural inflections, auxiliary verbs in English) is also essential so that the sentences sound 'grammatical' to native speakers. Models of sentence production have been proposed and they primarily describe how a canonical sentence is formulated through different stages of processing. There is not yet a model that discusses in detail how different sentence forms (e.g. active versus passive sentences, or full versus elliptical sentences) are selected. The following section will discuss one of the most popular sentence production models according to Garrett (1982, 1984) and an attempt will be made to link the model to some recent findings in discourse. Data from two groups of Cantonese agrammatic subjects identified by a cluster analysis procedure will then be presented. The extensive use of elliptical sentences by these Cantonese agrammatic subjects is interpreted as a possible compensatory strategy. Then a concluding remark will be made to highlight the limitations in using models of normal language processing to explain symptoms of aphasic people and vice versa.

## A model of sentence production

The sentence production model based on Garrett (1982; 1984) and further expanded by Bock (1987), LaPointe and Dell (1989), and Schwartz (1987) is probably the most influential model proposed to date. This model characterises sentence production as a sequence of processing stages.

To illustrate the processes involved in this model, Figure 9.1 shows the processes involved in formulating the sentence 'the boy is kicking the ball'. In order to construct this sentence, the 'non-linguistic message' triggers a search through the mental lexicon (Garrett, 1982, 1984). The search will yield three lexical items, 'boy', 'kick' and 'ball'. The lexical items generated are still in their abstract forms. They do not have the phonetic representations. At this stage, a functional or predicate–argument structure is also formulated. This structure specifies that there will be two nouns (an agent and an object) and a verb (action) involved. The form of this argument structure is also in its abstract form, that is, the order of the elements in this structure is not yet determined. A third operation that takes place is the assignment of the lexical items (i.e. 'boy', 'kick' and 'ball') to roles within the predicate–argument structure. These three operations give rise to a representation that carries information as to who-does-what-to-whom (Schwartz, 1987).

In the next processing stage, the phonological representations of the lexical items are retrieved whereas the surface sentence frame is also determined. In this example, an active sentence is selected at the planning frame. A further operation will involve slotting the three lexical items with their phonological forms in the sentence frame with the insertion of function words such as article, auxiliary verb and the 'ing'

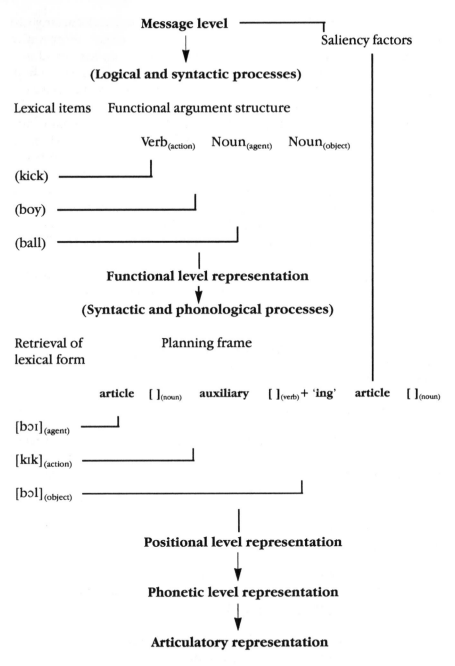

**Figure 9.1** Model of sentence production according to Garrett

inflection. With these syntactic and phonological processes, a positional level representation is created. Precise production is achieved (articulatory level representation) after the phonetic rules are applied (phonetic level representation).

This model describes primarily the formulation of canonical word order, i.e. SVO in English (e.g. The boy is kicking the ball). However, it does not specify what determines the choice between canonical and non-canonical structures such as passive (The ball is kicked by the boy) or elliptical sentences ('kicking the ball' in a discourse chain where the subject (i.e. 'the boy') is understood). There is some evidence that the choice between sentence structures is affected by pragmatic and discourse considerations (Berndt, 1991). Cross-language psycholinguistic studies have identified at least three saliency factors: the recency effect in a discourse; the motivation of the speaker; or the emphasis that the speaker wants to put (Sridhar, 1988). It is not yet clear how these factors fit into the sentence production model described above. However, it is likely that they operate directly between the message level and the processing stage where the sentence frame is formed (Figure 9.1).

The following section will present data to show the extent of elliptical sentences being produced by Cantonese normal and agrammatic speakers in a narrative task.

## Data from Cantonese agrammatic speakers

### Subjects

A group of 30 monolingual Cantonese-speaking aphasic subjects and 10 non-aphasic subjects participated in this study. The experimental group (aphasic subjects) and the control group (non-aphasic subjects) were not significantly different in age (Mann–Whitney $U = 130.5, p > 0.5$) or years of education (Mann–Whitney $U = 136.5, p > 0.6$). All the aphasic subjects had a left hemisphere stroke and were at least one month post stroke.

### Procedures

Subjects were asked to describe four sets of sequenced pictures used by Menn and Obler's (1990) cross-linguistic study of agrammatism. The theme of each set of sequenced pictures was:

1.   a farmer planting and harvesting a crop (four pictures),
2.   a thief being caught in a burglary attempt (four pictures),
3.   a picnicking young couple whose barbecue meat is being stolen by a dog (four pictures), and
4.   a man who has overslept is woken by his wife, and falls asleep at his office (five pictures).

All the narratives were videotaped and were later transcribed and segmented into propositional utterances according to the procedures described by Saffran, Berndt and Schwartz (1989). All neologism, repairs and repetitions were excluded from the propositional utterances.

Analysis was then carried out on the extracted propositional utterances with the following structures counted:

1. the number of morphemes
2. the number of function (closed class) words
3. the number of complete sentences (a complete sentence contains at least a subject and a main verb)
4. the number of embedded sentences (an embedded sentence contains two or more clauses)
5. the number of elliptical sentences (a sentence was considered to be elliptical for the purpose of this study if the pre-verbal noun phrase, based on the context of the pictures, was omitted)

These structures represented the sentence length, morphology and complexity of the propositional utterances. From these, the mean length of utterance (MLU), the proportion of closed class words, the proportion of complete sentences, the proportion of embedded sentences, and the proportion of elliptical sentences were calculated for each subject.

Cluster analysis was then carried out using these calculated production measures to combine individual aphasic subjects to form relatively homogeneous clusters based on their similarity. An agglomerative hierarchical cluster analysis using the average linkage method on the converted z-scores of the production measures (Norusis, 1986) was employed.


## Results

Three major clusters (plus three outliers) resulted from the analysis. The mean production measures of these three clusters and the control group are reported in Table 9.1. Mann–Whitney U-tests were carried out between the three aphasic groups and the control group on these measures to determine which aphasic group was significantly different from the control group. Two of the groups (Groups II and III) were clearly identified as agrammatic (see Table 9.1). They produced significantly shorter sentences, fewer closed class words, fewer complete and embedded sentences than the control group ($p < 0.05$). Furthermore, Group II produced significantly more elliptical sentences than the control group ($p < 0.05$) while the production of elliptical sentences by Group III was not significantly different from the control group.

**Table 9.1** Mean production measures of the aphasic groups and the control group

| | Aphasic group | | | Control |
| | I<br>N = 10 | II<br>N = 6 | III<br>N = 11 | N = 10 |
|---|---|---|---|---|
| Mean length of<br>utterance | 6.41<br>(1.03) | 2.44*<br>(0.36) | 3.95*<br>(0.70) | 7.02<br>(2.41) |
| Proportion of<br>closed class words | 0.55<br>(0.04) | 0.32*<br>(0.06) | 0.51*<br>(0.04) | 0.56<br>(0.04) |
| Proportion of<br>complete sentences | 0.41<br>(0.12) | 0.09*<br>(0.08) | 0.22*<br>(0.09) | 0.43<br>(0.16) |
| Proportion of<br>embedded sentences | 0.33<br>(0.09) | 0.04*<br>(0.06) | 0.13*<br>(0.08) | 0.40<br>(0.18) |
| Proportion of<br>elliptical sentences | 0.47<br>(0.12) | 0.91*<br>(0.07) | 0.68<br>(0.13) | 0.55<br>(0.15) |

\* Indicates significantly different from the control group at 0.05 level using Mann–Whitney U-test.

## Discussion

Both Groups II and III were clearly demonstrating features of agrammatism, characterised by shorter and simpler sentences with fewer morphological structures. The omission of morphological structures (i.e. the closed class words) in agrammatism has been interpreted as a disruption in one of the operations which creates the positional level of representation (Garrett, 1982, 1984; see Figure 9.1). However, there has not yet been any satisfactory explanation for the rarity of complex structures (e.g. embedded sentences) using the model. It may be argued that it is quite natural for an impaired speaker to resort to simpler structures available in his or her language. This was also reflected in the use of elliptical sentences. However, only Group II, but not Group III, used significantly more elliptical sentences than the control group. Group II had a more severe agrammatism than those in Group III. Hence it appears that the more severe agrammatic group resorted to using more elliptical sentences as part of the process of simplifying and shortening their sentences.

    As discussed earlier, the saliency factors operating between the message level and the processing stage where the surface sentence structure is formulated determines the type of sentence to be selected. The present data only showed that the more severe group (Group II) used elliptical sentences more extensively than the control group. These data suggest that the saliency factors were operating to adapt to the agrammatism by selecting the elliptical structures, which the speakers might find easier to produce because they are simpler, shorter and acceptable in Cantonese discourse. It may well be that the subjects had a restriction in their capacity to process complex grammatical structures. This forced them to use the simpler structures. In other words, it is suggested that the frequent use of elliptical sentences is a symptom of the adaptation rather than a product of the impairment. This view is also shared by Stemberger (1985), who argued that aphasic speakers could only produce the simplest, and most frequent forms of grammatical structures.

Kolk and Heeschen (1990) review their series of studies which have investigated this impairment–adaptation dichotomy in agrammatic subjects. They conclude that the adaptation hypothesis offers an account for agrammatism, dysprosody, low speech rate, and reduced variety of grammatical form. Kolk and Heeschen (1990) also suggest that the communicative situation plays a role in whether the aphasic person opts to use a compensatory strategy. For example, an agrammatic speaker may not opt to use telegraphic speech in formal situations but may choose to use simpler structures which require less correction when a listener is impatient. This task-dependency was investigated by Hofstede and Kolk (1994), Heeschen (1985) and Martin, Wetzel, Blossom-Stach and Feher (1989). It was found that there were changes in the agrammatic speech in both picture description and free conversations suggesting that agrammatic patients have the ability to adapt to the communicative context. Since our data were based on connected speech in describing pictures, it may well be that the agrammatic subjects in this study were fully exploiting the inherent characteristics of Cantonese, that is, to use elliptical sentences extensively once the topic was understood in the context.

Kolk and Heeschen (1990) also suggest that adaptation symptoms are not always present because it is optional rather than mandatory. However, we believe that the compensation, if it exists, is severity-dependent rather than an option. The more severe agrammatic patients must adapt more because they have less linguistic structures in which to send their message or be part of a conversation. The optionality allows for an easy explanation for the variable symptoms in individuals. However, it is cognitively demanding for an individual to exercise control over such options. Our data, with the more severe group producing more elliptical sentences, lend support to the severity-dependent hypothesis.

The data presented here are suggestive but not conclusive of whether the extensive use of elliptical sentences is a product of the impairment or a symptom of adaptation. For this to be clarified, an experimental design is needed to examine whether agrammatic speakers still produce elliptical sentences when the topic or subject is obligatory. If the speakers, who produced extensive elliptical sentences in narratives, produce only a few elliptical sentences under obligatory situations, the cause is more of a compensatory strategy. If, however, elliptical sentences are produced in both tasks, this could be a reflection of the impairment.

## Conclusion

This chapter has briefly reviewed the issue of compensation at a neuro-biological and at a symptom level. It has presented data from a linguistic study in Cantonese which suggests that compensation occurs in the form of an increased number of elliptical sentences in Cantonese agrammatic subjects. If impaired individuals use a great deal of compensation, it is difficult to attribute abnormal symptoms in impaired individuals simply as evidence of the breakdown of normal language processing. In addition, using data from normal individuals to determine the level of breakdown in impaired individuals will be complicated by the compensatory strategies of the impaired individual. This has led to the current situation in which symptoms of impaired individuals are described as heterogeneous and not easily explained by models of normal language processing. However, this is not to suggest that models cannot be used to explain the symptomatology of the language impaired patient. It does argue, however, that researchers and clinicians alike must remain open to the possibility of compensation occurring at all levels of impairment, disability and handicap.

## Acknowledgements

The authors wish to thank Associate Professor Randi Martin, Associate Professor Kim Kirshner and Dr Kathryn Hird for comments on the early draft of this chapter.

The first author would also like to thank the Department of Speech and Hearing Science, Curtin University for providing financial support during the preparation of this chapter.

## References

Berndt, R.S. (1991). Sentence processing in aphasia. In M.T. Sarno (Ed.) *Acquired Aphasia*, 2nd edn. New York: Academic Press.

Bock, K. (1987). Coordinating words and syntax in speech plans. In A> Ellis (Ed.) *Progress in the Psychology of Language*, Vol. 3. London: Erlbaum.

Flohr, H. (Ed.) (1988) *Post-lesion Neural Plasticity*. Berlin: Springer-Verlag.

Garrett, M.F. (1982). Production of speech: Observations from normal and pathological language use. In A.W. Ellis (Ed.) *Normality and Pathology in Cognitive Functions*. London: Academic Press.

Garrett, M.F. (1984). The organisation of processing structure for language production: Applications to aphasic speech. In D. Caplan, A.R. Lecours and A. Smith (Eds) *Biological Perspectives on Language*. Cambridge: MIT Press.

Halliday, M.A.K. (1985). *An Introduction to Functional Grammar*. London: Edward Arnold.

Heeschen, C. (1985). Agrammatism and paragrammatism: A fictitious opposition. In M.L. Kean (Ed.) *Agrammatism*. Orlando: Academic Press.

Hofstede, B.T.M. and Kolk, H.H.J. (1994). The effects of task variation on the production of grammatical morphology in Broca's aphasia: A multiple case study. *Brain and Language*, 46, 278–328.

Kertesz, A. (1982). *The Western Aphasia Battery*. New York: Grune and Stratton.

Kolk, H. and Heeschen, C. (1990) Adaptation symptoms and impairment symptoms in Broca's aphasia. *Aphasiology*, 4 (3), 221–231.

Kolk, H. and van Grunsven, M.J.F. (1985). Agrammatism as a variable phenomenon. *Cognitive Neuropsychology*, 2(4), 347–384.

LaPointe, S.G. and Dell, G.S. (1989). A synthesis of some recent work in sentence production. In G.N. Carlson and M.K. Tanenhaus (Eds) *Linguistic Structure in Language Processing*. Dordrecht: Kluwer Academic.

Li, C.N. and Thompson, S.A. (1981). *Mandarin Chinese: A Functional Reference Grammar*. Berkeley: University of California Press.

Martin, R.C., Wetzel, W.F., Blossom-Stach, C. and Feher, E (1989). Syntactic loss versus processing deficit: An assessment of two theories of agrammatism and syntactic comprehension deficits. *Cognition*, 32, 157–191.

Menn, L. and Obler, L.K. (Eds) (1990). *Agrammatic Aphasia: A Cross-Language Narrative Sourcebook*. Amsterdam: John Benjamins.

Norusis, M.J. (1986). *SPSS/PC+ Advance Statistics*. Chicago: SPSS Inc.

Packard, J. (1990). Agrammatism in Chinese: A case study. In L. Menn and L.K. Obler. (Eds) *Agrammatic Aphasia: A Cross-Language Narrative Sourcebook*. Amsterdam: John Benjamins.

Saffran, E.M., Berndt, R.S. and Schwartz, M.F. (1989). The quantitative analysis of agrammatic production: procedure and data. *Brain and Language*, 37, 440–479.

Schwartz, M.F. (1987). Patterns of speech production deficits within and across aphasia syndromes: Application of a psycholinguistic model. In M. Coltheart, G. Sartori and R. Job, (Eds) *The Cognitive Neuropsychology of Language*. London: Lawrence Erlbaum.

Seron, X. (1984). Reeducation strategies in neuropsychology: cognitive and pragmatic approaches. In F.C. Rose (Ed.) *Advances in Neurology*, 42. Raven Press: New York.

Sridhar, S.N. (1988). *Cognition and sentence production: A Cross-linguistic Study*. New York: Springer-Verlag.

Stemberger, J.P. (1985). Bound morpheme loss errors in normal and agrammatic speech: One mechanism or two. *Brain and Language*, 25, 246–256

Tsao, F-F. (1990). *Sentence and clause structure in Chinese: A Functional Perspective*. Taipei: Student Book.

World Health Organization (1980). *International Classification of Impairment, Disability and Handicap*. Geneva: WHO.

# Synthesis

Most people will experience the effects of a communication difficulty during their lifetime. Some will care for a parent with dementia or a child with unintelligible speech. Others will become hard of hearing as they age, or suffer a stroke that will leave them unable to express their wants and needs clearly. A significant number of children have difficulty learning to read and spell and that limits their academic achievement and employment potential. The role of speech–language pathologists is to assess communication difficulties and implement intervention to ameliorate their effects. Successful intervention is inextricably linked to the body of knowledge that characterises the nature of the many different types of communication impairment.

As with any body of research literature, however, there is ambiguity, contradiction and deficiencies. Researchers approach the study of communication impairment with questions and methodologies that are formed by their discipline whether it be neurophysiology, linguistics, psychology, psycholinguistics or speech–language pathology. Each discipline has its own set of assumptions that are reflected in the content of the chapters in this book. In this final chapter we attempt to make a synthesis of the contributors' different perspectives of the problem addressed by the workshop: the extent to which studies of normal language can inform models of language impairment; and how the study of language impairment illuminates normal language function.

Our expectation of consensus was not high, given the range of disciplines represented and the variety of aspects of language examined. Nevertheless three conclusions were evident.

- Studies of impaired individuals have made a crucial contribution to our current understanding of normal speech and language function.
- Methodological issues continue to cloud the reported differences between normal and impaired individuals.

• Interpreting data from impaired individuals always involves making theoretical assumptions that constrain their usefulness in characterising non-impaired mental processing.

## Advances in understanding normal function

The first three chapters provide clearcut examples of research studies affirming the notion that the nature of normal language function can be adduced from the behaviour of people with disordered communication. Coltheart argues that the study of aphasic language has yielded a multitude of results that provide indisputable support for the general architecture of a model for reading. While two routes to reading can be independently damaged, they may generate interesting patterns of sparing and impairment that can only be understood once real-time computational modelling is used. This model has benefited our understanding of acquired reading disorders and pointed the way for the effective treatment of acquired dyslexia. McCormack shows that prosody may not be an independently functioning module of language. That is, prosody is so intertwined with other functions of language that it is rarely disordered without an accompanying impairment in speech, syntax or lexical processing. Butcher applies a novel approach. He examined speech disordered children's response to treatment and used these data to evaluate models of speech processing. The findings bear on current concerns in computational modelling of language, that is, the conditions under which a modular process can be 'tipped' into adequate functioning. These three examples demonstrate different ways in which the study of impaired individuals can advance our understanding of normal language function. Without such studies of impairment, our knowledge of normal function would be impoverished.

## Methodological issues

Nevertheless, it became clear that there was general consensus about the need to examine critically some of the procedures commonly used in studies of impaired and normal language. Two aspects of methodology received detailed examination. The first concerned the definition of 'normal' and individual variation within the normal group. Dodd, So and Li (Chapter 6) provided data that demonstrated that bilingual people follow a different course of language acquisition than monolingual speakers of both their languages. Since more than 50% of the world's population is bilingual or trilingual, should monolingual English speakers' developmental path to speaking and reading be considered the norm? Further, Martin's review (Chapter 5) indicated that within the normal population, there are large individual differences in performance on tasks used to assess language function and cognition. The use of grouped normal data obscures these differences, casting doubt on the concept of 'normality' and making comparisons of 'normal' and impaired data problematic. Martin argued that, in some circumstances, case studies of normal subjects should be used rather than group studies.

The second concern related to the validity of the measurement tools used to study speech and language function. Kennedy (Chapter 8) reviewed critiques of standard language assessments. One problem with many language measures is that they use indirect assessment methods that are contaminated by non-linguistic factors (e.g. attention, perception, working memory and motor skills). Murdoch (Chapter 7) discussed the limitations of the models of subcortical participation in language that result from the inadequacies of the current neuro-imaging techniques such as CT and MRI. In agreement with Martin, Murdoch argued the need for future studies to focus first on case studies of normal rather than impaired subjects, applying functional brain imaging methods such as PET and SPECT.

Novel theoretical insights most often seem to follow advances in methodological procedures. Such advances are not only made through technological innovation but also depend upon re-examination of generally held methodological assumptions. Researchers focusing on impaired language have always been concerned with the issue of what is normal. It seems that there is now enough evidence to force reconsideration of how 'normality' is defined and assessed.

## Theoretical constraints imposed by assumptions

People with speech and language impairments are both neurobiologically and behaviourally different to normal subjects. Application of conclusions based on data from impaired function to normal function, and vice versa, therefore, need to be cautiously made. Campbell (Chapter 4) confronts this issue by focusing on people born profoundly hearing impaired and the variability in their language mastery. One of her important conclusions is that although language can be acquired, the type of language learned (e.g. Sign) influences not only cognition but also cortical functioning. Consequently, the relationship between the primary aetiology of a communication difference and measured behaviour might be more complex than is often assumed.

Kennedy (Chapter 8) reviews the range of assumptions that are implicit in much work that has investigated impaired function (e.g. subtractivity, transparency, modularity). She argues that while some of these assumptions can be supported, many pose inherently insurmountable obstacles to scientific examination of linguistic–cognitive functioning in both normal and impaired people. A concrete example of the difficulties inherent in the transparency and subtractivity assumptions is provided by Yiu and Worrall (Chapter 9). Their cross-linguistic study provides support for the adaptation hypothesis which holds that some symptoms of aphasia reflect patients' compensatory strategies rather than direct evidence concerning the effects of lesions. Yiu and Worrall concluded that there is a need to recognise issues such as compensation when evaluating models of language processing.

When researchers first began to employ designs that included groups of people with impairment they assumed that there was a relatively straightforward relationship between the type of impairment and the behaviour observed. Over the past few decades it has become clear that this is not so. There is a need, then, not only to define assumptions that have previously been implicit, but also to design studies that directly examine them.

## Conclusions

Understanding human language function is now a major research endeavour. The amount and variety of studies is growing rapidly. It is therefore timely to reflect on the validity of the methodologies used and the soundness of the implicit assumptions made. The themes discussed have implications for researchers who study impaired individuals to inform understanding of normal speech and language functions; for researchers who justify their research of speech and language function of normal individuals in terms of its long-term clinical applicability; and for clinicians who need to interpret both knowledge bases to implement appropriate intervention.

### Studies of impairment

Researchers who use data from impaired individuals to build theory of normal function need to be aware of the assumptions underlying their conclusions. Direct translation of evidence from impaired function to the description of normal function can only rarely be made.

### Studies of normality

Researchers studying people with no evidence of speech and language impairment need to consider what 'normal' can include. Many languages and language learning contexts have yet to be studied. Further, the performance of individuals within the normal range varies greatly, a point La Pointe emphasised, in the Introduction, by asking the question, 'When does dusk become night?', to draw attention to the continuum between normality and disorder.

## Clinical implications

Clinicians need to understand and interpret research studies of both normal and disordered speech and language. In seeking to ameliorate communication disorders, clinicians must use information from whatever source and attempt to discover the essence of a study's clinical applicability. Although there are a number of reasons why a particular treatment approach might fail, perhaps the most crucial is its theoretical rationale. A theoretical model that does not stand up to the rigours of clinical testing is doomed.

# Index